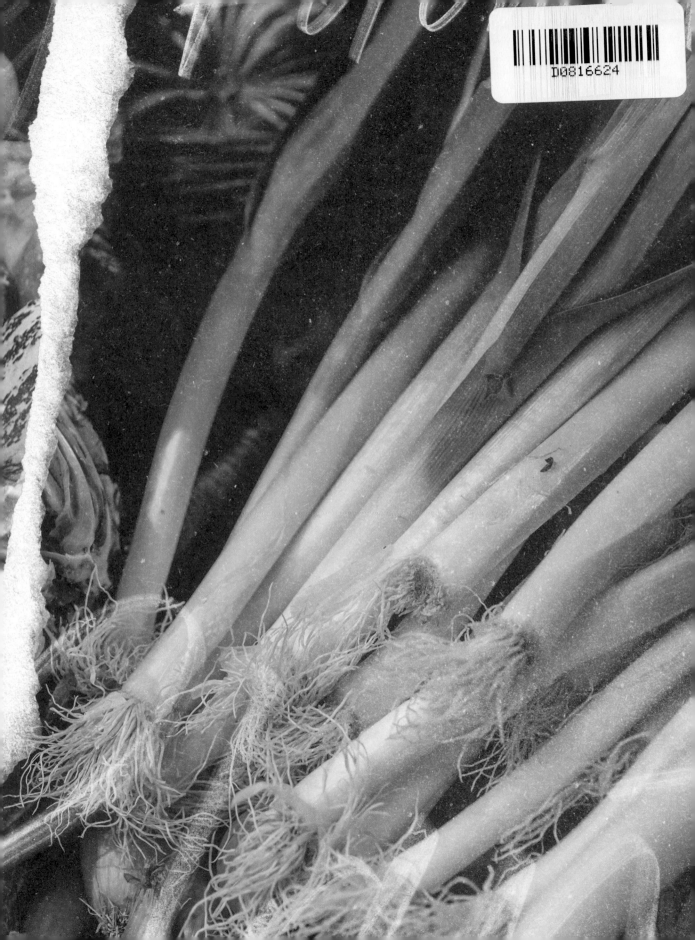

Plants Only Kitchen

Hardie Grant

QUADRILLE

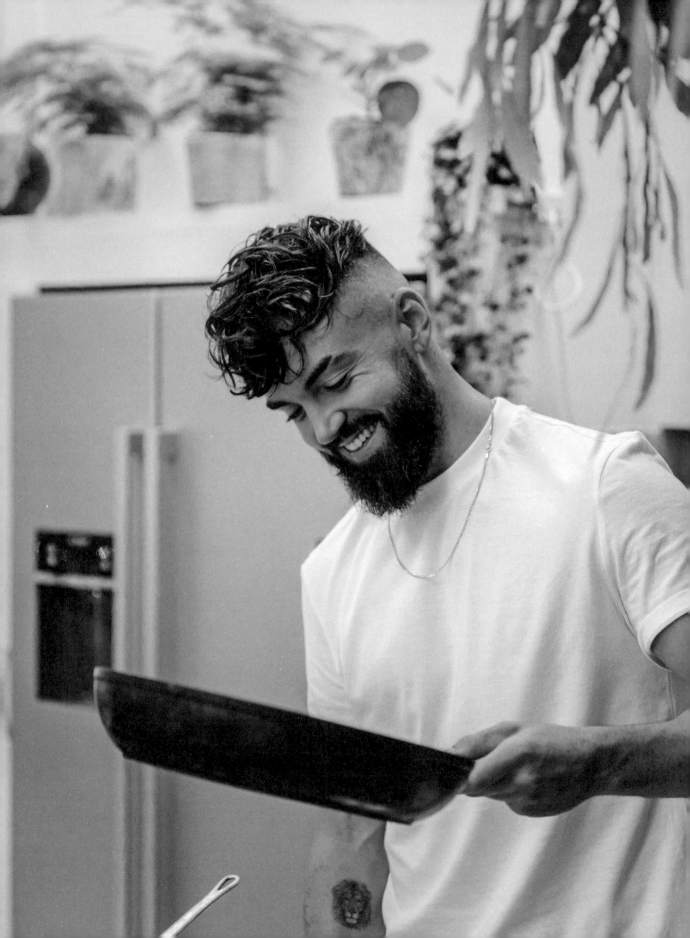

PLANTS ONLY KITCHEN

BY GAZ OAKLEY

OVER 70 DELICIOUS, SUPER SIMPLE, POWERFUL & PROTEIN-PACKED RECIPES FOR BUSY PEOPLE

Photography by Simon Smith
and Peter O'Sullivan

Hardie Grant

QUADRILLE

CONTENTS

07 BIG BAKES 130

08 BURGERS 146

09 VEGETABLES, SIDES & SALADS 158

10 DESSERTS 186

PLATE METHOD 213

INDEX & ACKNOWLEDGMENTS 216

KEY TO RECIPE ICONS

 #Gaz's15MinuteMeals

 One-pot Meal

 Protein-packed

 Can be made Gluten-free

 Gluten-free

 Meal Prep Star

 Batch Cooking

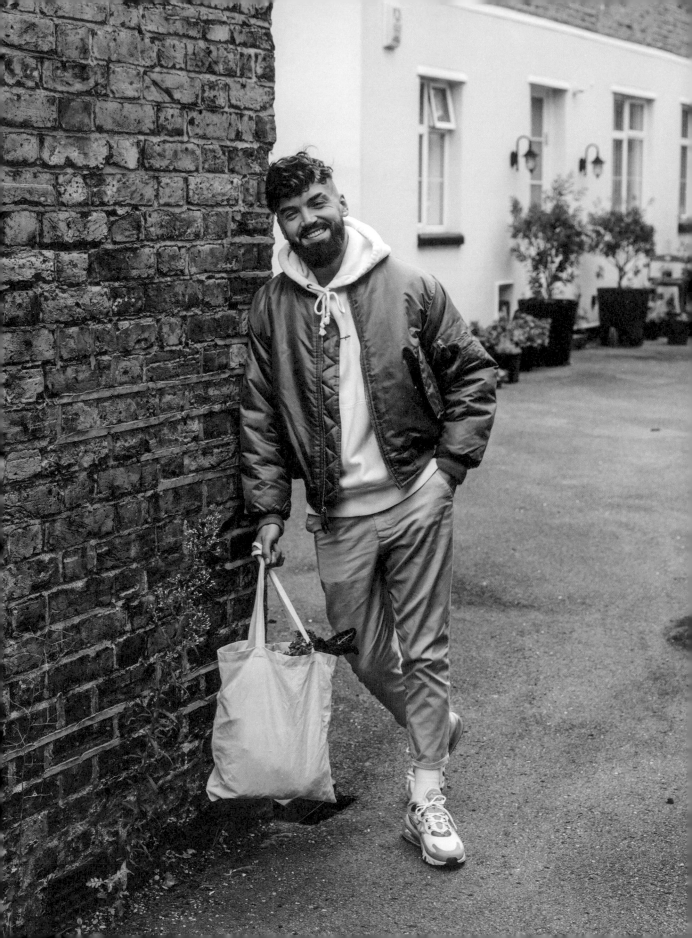

INTRODUCTION

Welcome to the plants only kitchen!

Wow... my third cookbook! I've worked on putting this book together over the last couple of years with the aim of creating beautiful tasty recipes that are SIMPLE to make. With no flair lost, these recipes will wow whoever you're cooking for.

I've made sure it's even easier for you by adding icons next to each recipe to let you know which ones are Protein-packed, Gluten-free, made in 15 minutes, good for Batch Cooking, a Meal Prep Star or a One-pot Meal (see Key on page 5). With these icons to help you, I hope you will find vegan cooking more accessible and satisfying than ever before. To make sure you are hitting all your nutritional needs, check out the Plate Method on page 213.

My passion for cooking is still as strong now, as when I first walked into a professional kitchen at 15 years old. I'm constantly learning and I love to experiment with new ingredients and techniques. You will see lots of dishes, ingredients and flavours in this book from all parts of the world, as I've been lucky enough to do a lot of travelling in recent years.

Every food picture in this book is real – there are no fancy food photography tricks – it is all real food, cooked and styled by me. I can guarantee that every dish tastes fantastic.

Whether you've just gone vegan, are trying to cut down on animal products or are a long-term vegan, I hope you will enjoy *Plants Only Kitchen*. I look forward to seeing your recreations!

Thanks so much for the support.

Love,

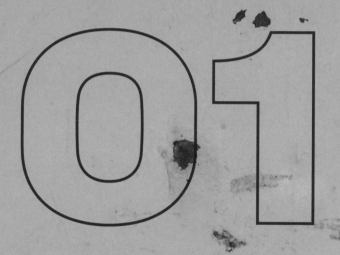

BREAK-FAST
Breakfast

PORRIDGE THREE WAYS

My go-to breakfast most days is porridge, but it can get boring. Here are my three favourite three ways to liven it up – they all taste amazing!

porridge base

45g (½ cup) porridge oats

240ml (1 cup) creamy non-dairy milk

2 tbsp maple syrup, or other natural sweetener

Add all the ingredients to a saucepan and place over a low heat.

Stir the porridge with a spatula for 4–5 minutes. Once the porridge is thick and creamy, remove from the heat and serve.

BANANA, HAZELNUT & CHOCOLATE

SERVES **1**	COOKS IN **10 MINS**	DIFFICULTY **3/10**

1 quantity of porridge base (above) with 3 tsp raw cacao powder added when cooking

1 tbsp coconut oil

1 banana, peeled and sliced lengthways

2 tsp coconut sugar

small handful of hazelnuts

1 tbsp cacao nibs

While your porridge base is cooking, place a non-stick frying pan (skillet) over a medium heat and add the coconut oil.

When the oil is hot, add the banana slices and sprinkle over the coconut sugar. Cook for 2 minutes on each side, until golden.

Top your chocolate porridge with the caramelized banana, hazelnuts and the cacao nibs.

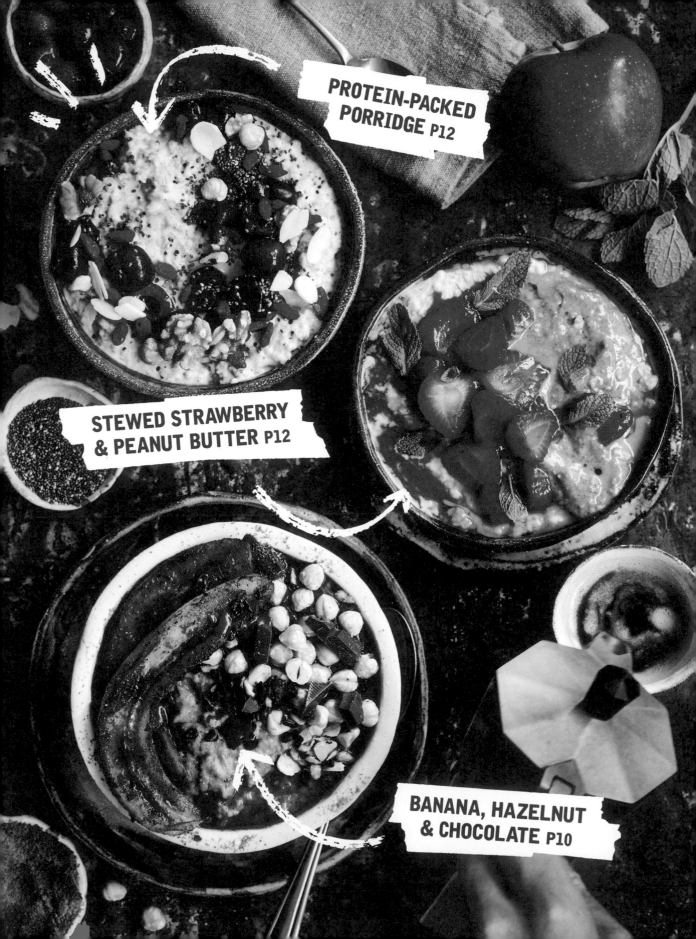

PROTEIN-PACKED PORRIDGE P12

STEWED STRAWBERRY & PEANUT BUTTER P12

BANANA, HAZELNUT & CHOCOLATE P10

STEWED STRAWBERRY & PEANUT BUTTER

SERVES **1**	COOKS IN **10 MINS**	DIFFICULTY **3/10**

6 strawberries, stems removed and halved

3 tbsp maple syrup

1 quantity of porridge base (page 10)

1 tbsp peanut butter (I recommend Pip & Nut maple)

fresh mint

First up, stew the strawberries. Put the strawberry halves into a saucepan with the maple syrup and a splash of water. Place over a low heat and cover.

Allow the strawberries to stew for around 8 minutes, while making your porridge base (page 10). Stir every now and then. Serve your porridge with the stewed strawberries, peanut butter and some fresh mint.

Pictured on page 11.

PROTEIN-PACKED PORRIDGE

SERVES **1**	COOKS IN **10 MINS**	DIFFICULTY **3/10**

1 quantity of porridge base (page 10)

100g (½ cup) cooked quinoa

2 tbsp hemp seeds

1 tbsp chia seeds

handful of mixed nuts

1 tbsp goji berries

handful of fresh cherries, de-stoned

Mix the cooked quinoa into your porridge base while it is cooking.

Top the quinoa porridge with the hemp seeds, chia seeds, mixed nuts, goji berries and cherries.

Pictured on page 11.

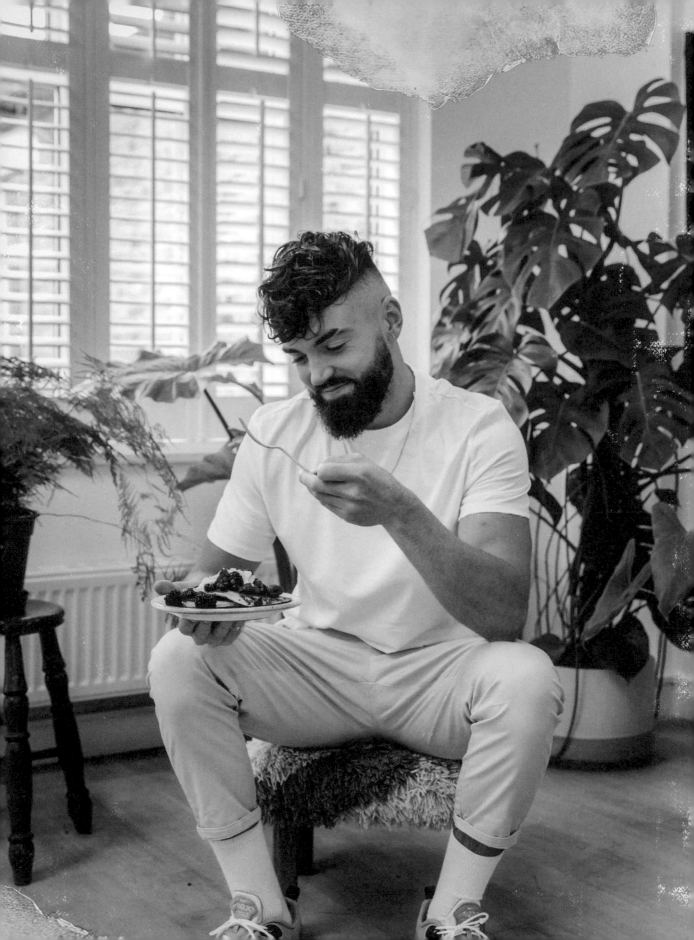

PROTEIN BLUEBERRY PANCAKES

Believe it or not, buckwheat is actually a fruit seed, and is closely related to rhubarb. Buckwheat flour is great for gluten-free baking and is perfect for making quick breakfast pancakes like these, which are packed with protein.

SERVES 2	COOKS IN 25 MINS	DIFFICULTY 3/10

120g (1 cup) buckwheat flour

1 tsp baking powder

25g (1 scoop) vegan protein powder

240–300ml (1–1¼ cups) non-dairy milk

3 tbsp agave nectar, or other natural sweetener

2 tbsp coconut oil, for frying

small handful of fresh blueberries

for the berry sauce

100g (1 cup) frozen mixed berries

juice of ½ lemon

to garnish

sprinkle of hemp seeds

2 tbsp non-dairy yogurt

fresh mint

drizzle of maple syrup (optional)

In a bowl, mix together the buckwheat flour, baking powder and protein powder. Whisk in 240ml (1 cup) milk and the sweetener. The batter should be slightly thick, but still pourable. Add a touch more non-dairy milk if needed. Set the batter aside.

To make the sauce, add the frozen berries and lemon juice to a small saucepan, and place over a very low heat. Cover and simply allow the berries to cook down for 10 minutes.

To cook the pancakes, place a non-stick frying pan (skillet) over a medium heat. Carefully, using kitchen paper, rub some of the coconut oil into the pan. When the pan is hot, ladle in a spoonful of the batter. Use the back of the ladle to spread the pancake out into a nice circular shape. Quickly drop in some of the fresh blueberries.

Cook the pancakes on each side for around 2 minutes or until golden. Repeat the process until you've used all the batter. To speed up the cooking, I like to get a couple of frying pans (skillets) going at the same time! Make sure you carefully grease the pans between cooking each pancake and turn down the heat if needed. I recommend using a palette knife to flip the pancakes.

Serve your pancakes with the berry sauce, a sprinkle of hemp seeds, a spoonful of non-dairy yogurt and some fresh mint.

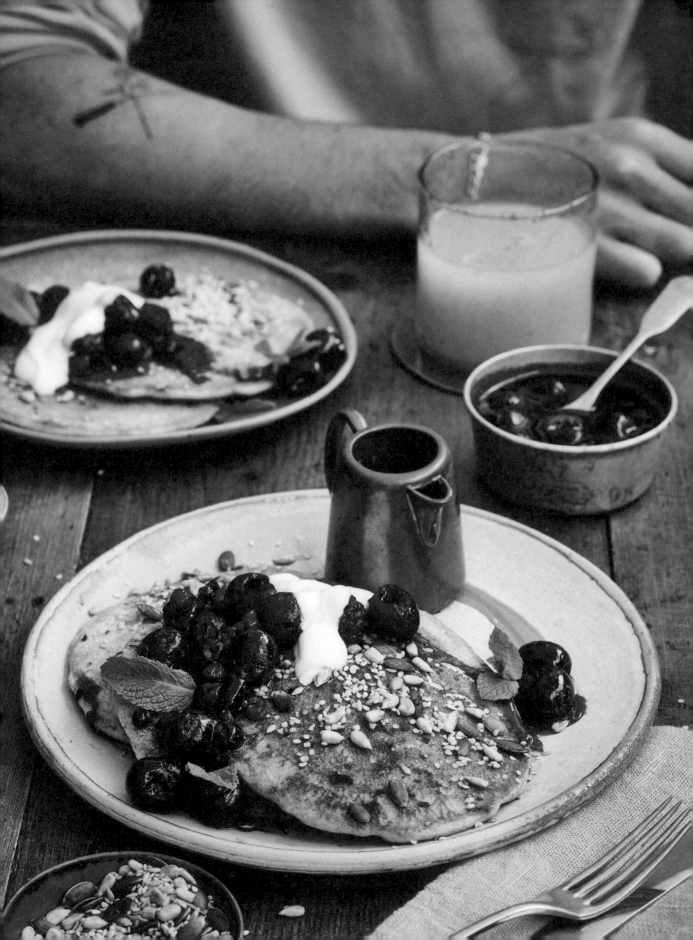

SCRAMBLED ACKEE

See how 'eggy' my Scrambled Ackee looks on page 20. Ackee is a Jamaican fruit, typically served with salt fish. It can be bought from most supermarkets in cans. It's incredibly creamy with a pleasant subtle flavour and with the addition of some spices, makes an epic scramble.

SERVES **4**	COOKS IN **20 MINS**	DIFFICULTY **3/10**

2 tbsp vegetable oil

5 spring onions (scallions), finely chopped

½ tsp dried garlic, or 1 fresh clove, finely chopped

½ yellow or red (bell) pepper, finely sliced

1 tsp smoked paprika

2 tsp dried thyme

1 x 540-g (19-oz) can ackee, drained and patted dry

60ml (¼ cup) non-dairy milk

handful of baby spinach leaves, washed, with any large stems removed

pinch ground pepper

pinch sea salt

Heat the oil in a non-stick frying pan (skillet) over a medium heat. Add the spring onions (scallions), garlic and sliced (bell) peppers. Sauté for 4 minutes or until softened.

Add the seasoning, with the paprika and thyme, then cook for a couple more minutes.

Add the ackee to the pan, then, using a wooden spoon, break the chunks up into small-sized pieces so it resembles scrambled eggs.

Cook the mixture for 4–5 minutes, stirring.

Turn the heat down to low, then add the milk. Gently stir over the heat for 2 minutes and then add the spinach.

Once the spinach has wilted, check the seasoning and serve.

Pictured on page 20.

MANGO BREAKFAST MUFFINS

I love these low sugar, grab-and-go muffins. They are easy to make and are great for kids! Feel free to experiment with the flavours by adding different dried or fresh fruits.

MAKES **8**	COOKS IN **50 MINS**	DIFFICULTY **5/10**

CAN BE GF

MEAL ☆ PREP

wet ingredients

1 over-ripe banana

360ml (1 ½ cups) soy milk, or non-dairy milk of your choice

115g (½ cup) vegan margarine, melted

2 tbsp chia seeds, blitzed to a fine powder

dry ingredients

120g (1 cup) plain (all-purpose) flour or gluten-free flour

3 tsp baking powder

100g (1 cup) ground oats or oat flour

50g (½ cup) ground almonds

100g (½ cup) coconut sugar

pinch sea salt

90g (½ cup) dried mango, finely chopped, plus extra for topping (optional)

Preheat your oven to 180°C (350°F). Line a muffin pan with 8 paper cases.

First up, prepare the wet mix by mashing the banana with the soy milk in a bowl. Once mashed (make sure there are minimal lumps), stir in the melted vegan margarine and the chia seeds.

Now for the dry ingredients. Sift the flour and baking powder into the bowl with the wet mix, then add the oats, almonds, sugar, salt and mango. Fold together.

Neatly spoon the batter into your muffin cases, filling each one about three-quarters full. Bake for 30 minutes. They should be risen and nicely golden brown. To test if they are cooked, insert a skewer into one of the muffins. If it comes out clean, they are done. If not, bake them a little longer.

Once baked, allow the muffins to cool slightly before serving. I like to garnish the top of the muffins with a few extra pieces of chopped mango.

If kept in an airtight container, the muffins will keep fresh for 2–3 days.

Pictured on page 19.

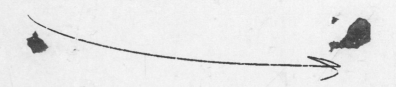

BOOST BARS

Another great grab-and-go recipe that will give you a real blast of energy. These can also be stored in a sealed container for up to 5 days, so you will always have a snack ready!

SERVES **12**	COOKS IN **30 MINS**	DIFFICULTY **3/10**

PRO TEIN GF MEAL ☆ PREP

180g (2 cups) rolled oats

60g (½ cup) mixed nuts, blitzed into small pieces

70g (½ cup) mixed seeds

3 tbsp raw cacao powder

4 tbsp shelled hemp seeds

4 tbsp chia seeds

25g (½ cup) goji berries, finely chopped

6 tbsp agave nectar

4 tbsp nut butter

for the topping

175g (1 cup) dark dairy-free chocolate, melted (optional)

Line a deep 23 x 23cm (9 x 9in) baking sheet with baking parchment and preheat your oven to 180°C (350°F).

Add all the ingredients, except the topping, to a large bowl and mix together using your hands.

Compact the mixture into your lined baking sheet, then place the tray into your oven and bake for 25 minutes. It should be firm to the touch and lightly coloured.

Once cooked, turn out onto a wire rack to cool. When cool, cut into 12 bars and drizzle with the melted dairy-free chocolate (if using).

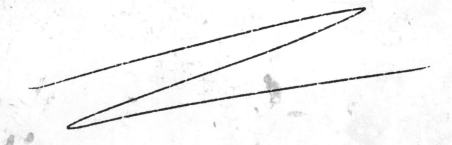

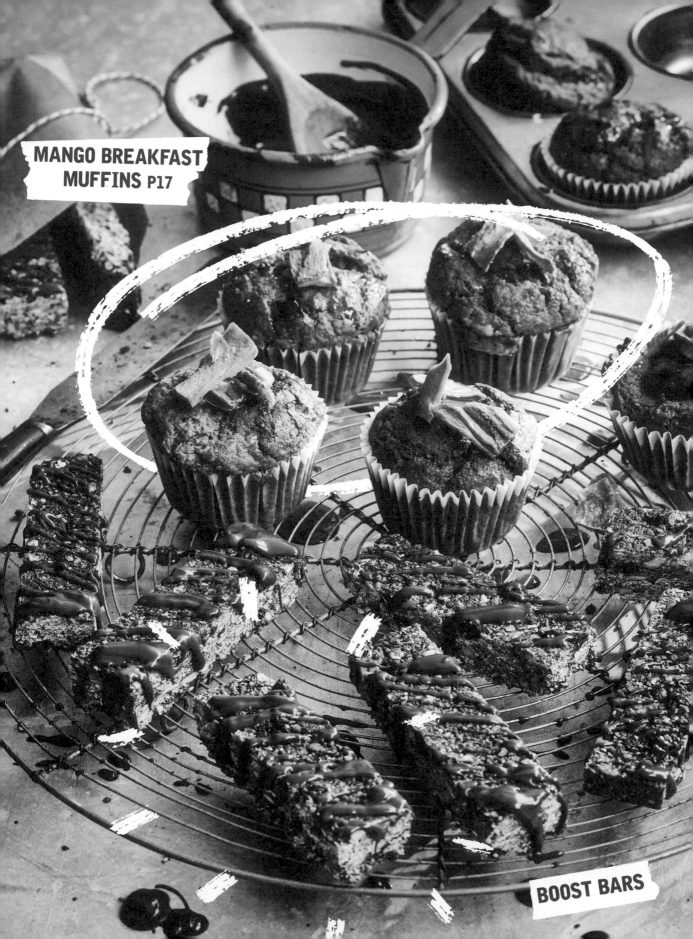

MANGO BREAKFAST MUFFINS P17

BOOST BARS

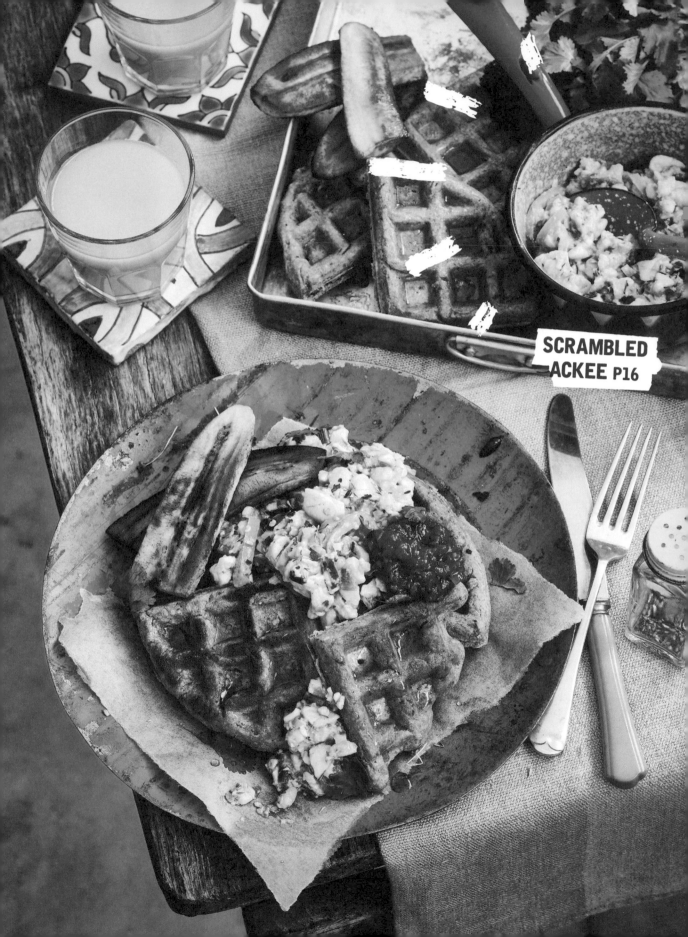

SCRAMBLED
ACKEE P16

CARIBBEAN WAFFLES

MAKES **2**	COOKS IN **35 MINS**	DIFFICULTY **5/10**

100g (1 cup) buckwheat flour

125g (1 cup) chickpea (gram) flour

2 tsp baking powder

1 tsp sea salt

1 tsp sweet smoked paprika

1 tsp dried thyme

1 tbsp jerk seasoning

240ml (1 cup) non-dairy milk

vegetable oil, for spraying

serve with

Scrambled Ackee (see page 16)

Fried Plantain (see page 169)

Combine all the dry ingredients in a mixing bowl, then whisk in the milk until there are no lumps and the mixture has a thick, batter-like consistency.

Set the batter aside to rest for at least 10 minutes.

Preheat your waffle machine to a medium heat and spray with a little oil.

Ladle in half of the mixture, then close the waffle machine. Allow the waffle to cook for 7 minutes at medium heat. Do not open the waffle machine during this time.

After 7 minutes, turn up the heat to high, and cook for a further 4 minutes.

Remove the waffle and repeat with the remaining mixture. Serve with Scrambled Ackee and Fried Plantain.

Oil in a spray bottle works really well for waffle machines.

GRIDDLE PAN WAFFLES
with Berry Compote

SERVES 4	COOKS IN **25 MINS**	DIFFICULTY **5/10**

for the waffles

1 ripe banana

480ml (2 cups) creamy non-dairy milk

3 tbsp maple syrup

2 tsp vanilla essence

1 tbsp chia seeds

260g (2 cups) self-raising flour or gluten-free self-raising flour

2 tsp baking powder

pinch sea salt

2 tbsp vegetable oil

for the compote

200g (2 cups) frozen mixed berries, defrosted

2 tbsp water

2 tbsp coconut sugar

1 tbsp fresh lemon juice

serve with

2 tbsp vegan yogurt

fresh mint

drizzle of maple syrup

Add the banana, milk, maple syrup and vanilla essence to a mixing bowl. Using a potato masher, mash the banana as much as you can to remove the lumps, then stir in the chia seeds.

Sift the flour, baking powder and salt into the banana mixture, then gently fold everything together using a spatula. Don't overmix or your waffle won't be light and fluffy when it's cooked.

Preheat a non-stick oven-proof griddle pan over a low heat and preheat your grill (broiler) to high.

Add the oil to the griddle pan, and when it's hot, add enough batter to cover the base of the pan. Use a spatula to help spread the batter into the corners of the pan.

Allow the waffle to cook for 4–5 minutes before placing the pan under the grill (broiler), on the bottom shelf, for 10 minutes.

While the waffle is cooking, add the compote ingredients to a saucepan. Place the pan over a low heat to bubble away until you're ready to serve, stirring occasionally.

After 10 minutes under the grill (broiler), your waffle should have risen nicely and be lovely and golden on top.

Top the waffle with the compote and serve with yogurt, fresh mint and maple syrup.

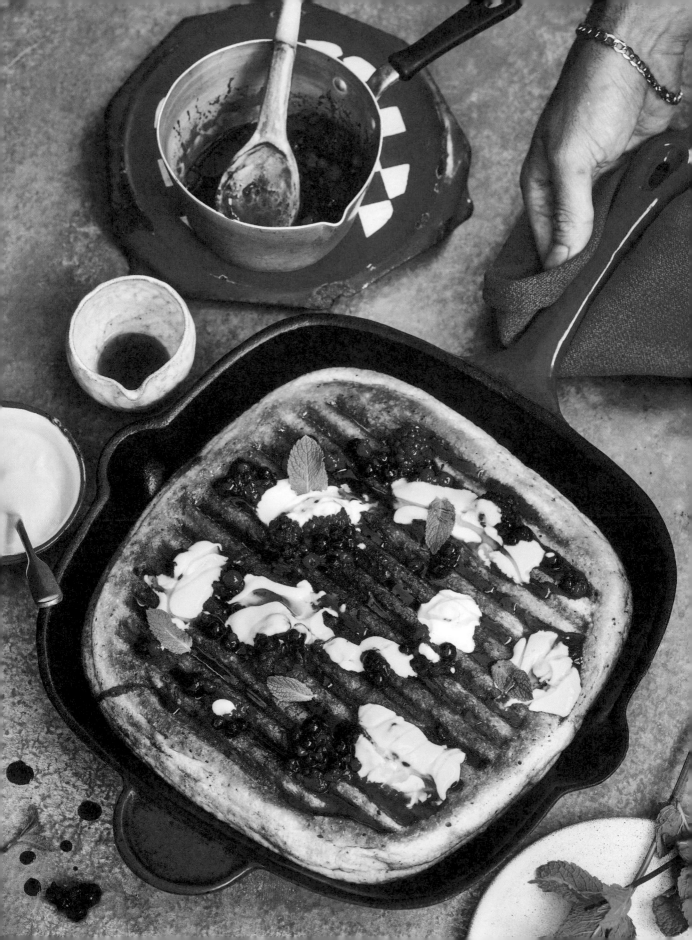

TEMPEH BACON BAGELS

Tempeh is one of my favourite vegan protein sources, try to find an organic version if you can. Tempeh is made from fermented soy beans, and because the whole bean is used, the protein content is high and the flavour is maximized. This quick 'bacon' glaze will take your tempeh to the next level.

SERVES **2**	COOKS IN **15 MINS**	DIFFICULTY **3/10**

vegetable oil, for frying

1 x 200-g (7-oz) block of tempeh, thinly sliced widthways

12 cherry tomatoes, on the vine

for the sticky glaze

2 tbsp maple syrup

2 drops of liquid smoke (optional)

¼ tsp smoked paprika

1 tbsp soy sauce or tamari

serve with

4 wholemeal bagels, toasted

fresh spinach leaves

vegan cream cheese

tomato ketchup

sprinkling of mixed seeds

Mix together the glaze ingredients in a small bowl.

Place a non-stick frying pan (skillet) over a medium heat. Add a little oil, followed by the tempeh slices. Cook the tempeh for 3 minutes on each side, brushing with the glaze on both sides.

Once the tempeh bacon is caramelized and sticky, remove from the pan and set the slices aside to crisp up.

Give the pan a quick wipe with kitchen paper before adding a touch more oil, then the cherry tomatoes. Just let them slightly blister in the pan for a couple of minutes.

Serve the tempeh bacon in toasted wholemeal bagels with the blistered tomatoes, some fresh spinach, vegan cream cheese, ketchup and a sprinkling of mixed seeds.

Liquid smoke is a great flavour enhancer. It adds a rich BBQ, smoky flavour to dishes.

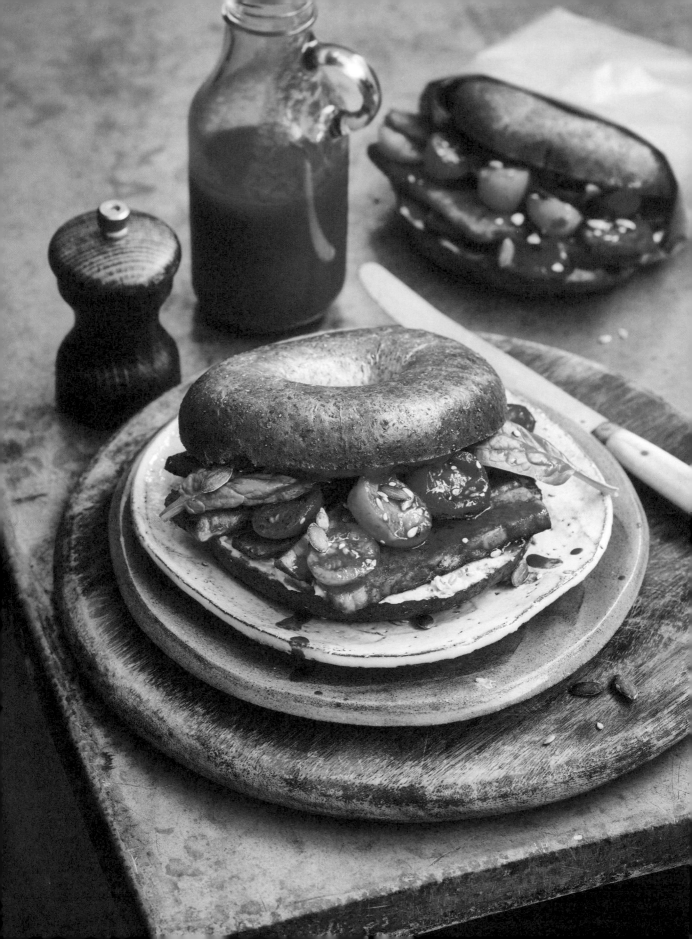

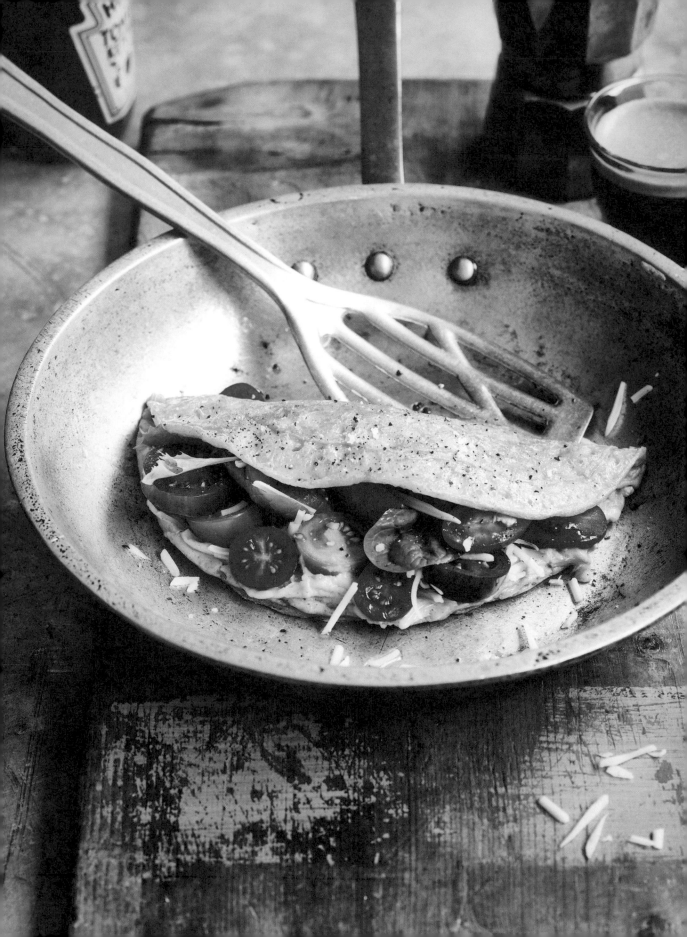

FLUFFY FRENCH STYLE OMELETTE

Looks like an omelette, tastes like an omelette and is made in no time at all!
Serve your omelette with a tasty filling of your choice.

SERVES **2**	COOKS IN **25 MINS**	DIFFICULTY **5/10**

1 x 280-g (10-oz) block tofu, patted dry

5 tbsp chickpea (gram) flour, or more as needed

1 tsp baking powder

½ tsp ground turmeric

½ tsp Kala Namak (optional)

½ tsp onion powder

1 tsp sea salt

1 tsp ground pepper

180ml (¾ cup) non-dairy milk

vegetable oil, for frying

filling suggestion

mixed tomatoes and salad leaves with grated vegan cheese

Add all the ingredients apart from the oil to a blender and blend until completely smooth. The mixture should be thick but pourable. If your mixture is for some reason too runny, add a little more chickpea (gram) flour.

Preheat a non-stick frying pan (skillet) over a medium heat and add a touch of oil. When hot, add enough of the tofu mixture to cover the base of the pan. Use the back of a ladle to spread the mixture out. Let the omelette cook for 3 minutes before carefully flipping over with a palette knife.

Cook for another 3 minutes before adding your chosen filling to the middle of the omelette. Carefully fold the omelette over to enclose the filling, remove from the pan and serve.

Kala Namak, also known as Himalayan Black Salt, gives the omelette a nice eggy taste.

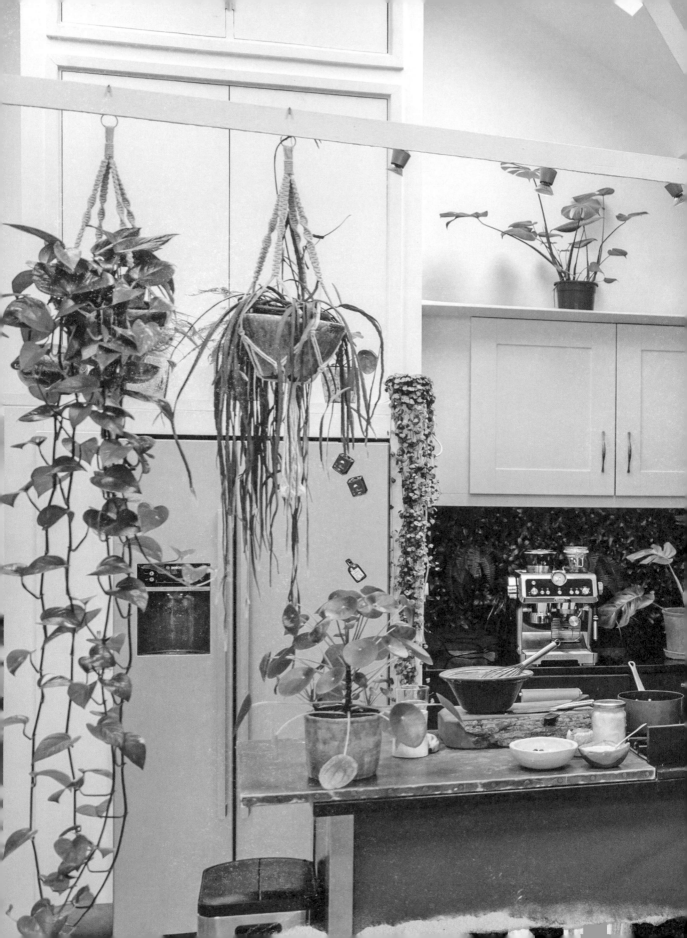

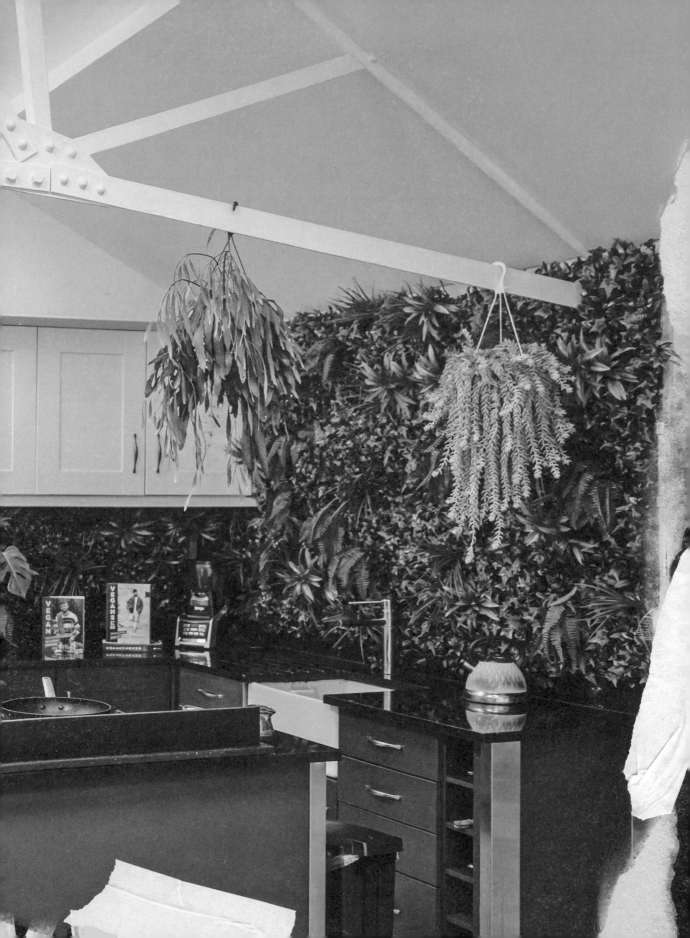

02

Soups

SOUPS

FRENCH ONION SOUP

| SERVES **4** | COOKS IN **65 MINS** | DIFFICULTY **3/10** |

2 tbsp vegan margarine

2 tbsp olive oil

4 banana shallots,
halved then finely sliced

3 large white onions,
halved then finely sliced

2 red onions, halved then
finely sliced

3 tsp sea salt

black pepper

1 tbsp fresh thyme leaves, plus
extra for serving

2 tsp dried sage

1 tbsp plain (all-purpose) flour
or gluten-free flour

240ml (1 cup) vegan-friendly
dry white wine

35ml (1 shot) brandy

1 litre (1¾ pints) hot
vegetable stock

1 bay leaf

1 rosemary sprig

4–6 slices of French baguette
(day-old bread works best)

1 garlic clove

grated vegan cheese

First up, place a large heavy-based saucepan over a low heat, then add the margarine and olive oil.

When hot, add the shallots and onions with the salt, pepper, thyme and sage. Allow the onions to sweat down and caramelize, this should take approximately 15–20 minutes. At first, it may look as though there are way too many onions in the pan, but after a little while they will shrink right down. Stir the onions often.

When the onions are beautiful and golden, add the flour and stir well to coat the onions. Cook out the flour for a minute or so before deglazing the pan with the white wine and the brandy. Bring the liquid to a boil before adding the hot vegetable stock, bay leaf and rosemary. Place a lid on the pan and let the soup cook away for 15–20 minutes.

Preheat your grill (broiler) to high.

Toast your slices of baguette. Cut the garlic clove in half and rub the cut side on each side of the slices of toasted bread.

Remove the bay leaf and rosemary sprig, then ladle the soup into your serving bowls and float a slice or two of toasted baguette on the surface of the soup in each bowl. Top each slice of baguette with a handful of the grated vegan cheese. Place your bowls onto a flat baking sheet then place each one under the grill (broiler) for 2 minutes.

Once the cheese has melted and is nice and golden, sprinkle over a few fresh thyme leaves, grind over some black pepper and serve up.

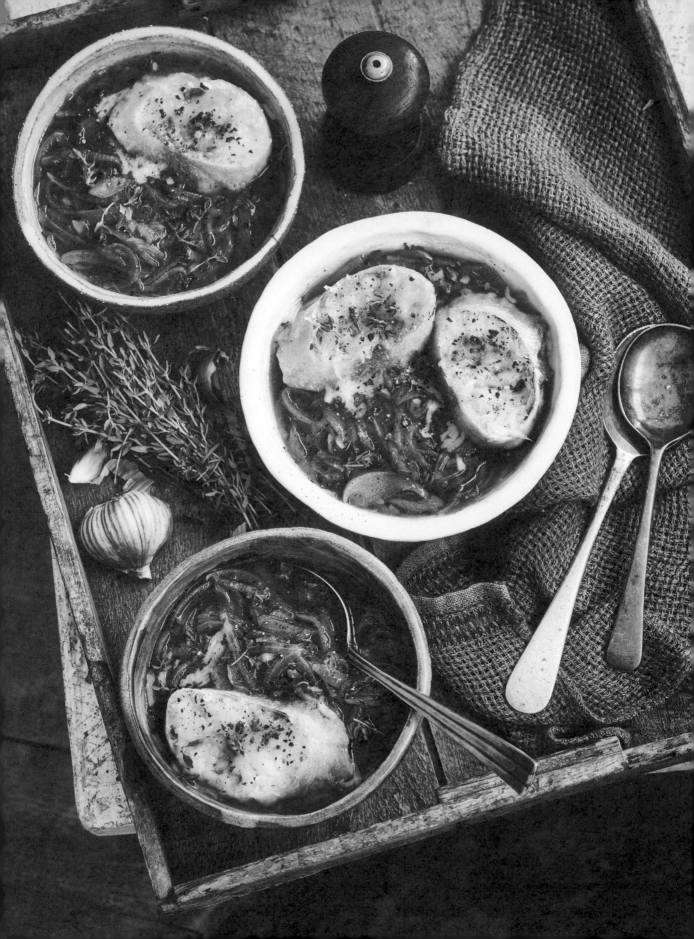

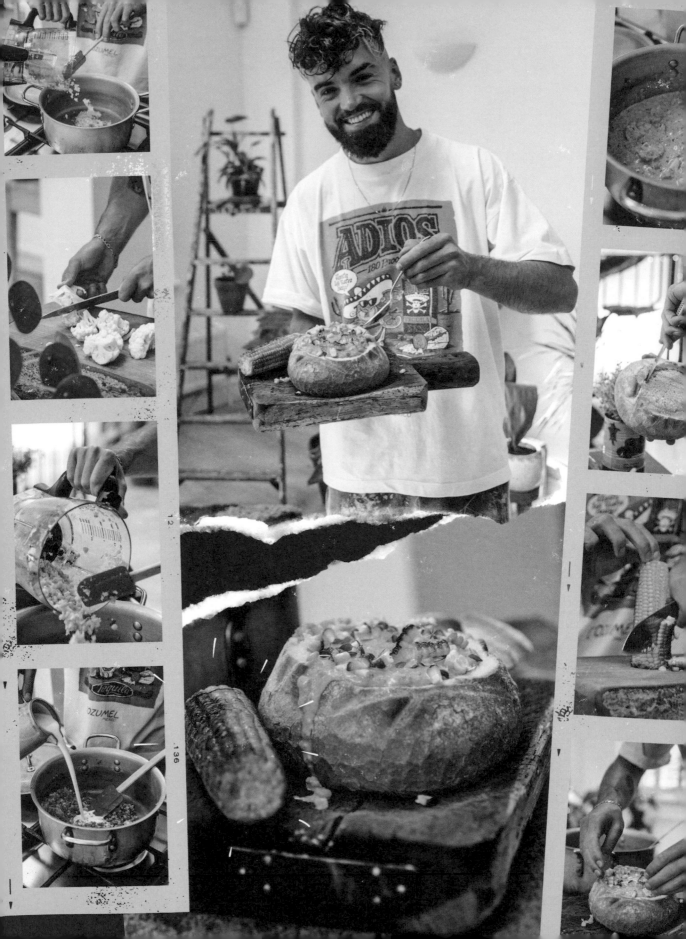

CHEAT'S CORN CHOWDER IN BREAD BOWL

SERVES **4**	COOKS IN **15 MINS**	DIFFICULTY **3/10**

1 onion, roughly chopped

2 celery sticks, roughly chopped

1 red chilli

3 garlic cloves

2 tbsp olive oil

1 tsp sweet smoked paprika

1 tbsp dried thyme

1 bay leaf

3 tbsp plain (all-purpose) flour

230ml (1 cup) vegan cream

480ml (2 cups) hot vegetable stock

560g (4 cups) sweetcorn, blitzed to a puree

2 Charred Corn cobs (page 183)

1 tbsp soy sauce or tamari

1 tsp sea salt

2 tsp black pepper

90g (1 cup) vegan cheese, grated (optional)

serve with

round loaf of bread, top cut off and middle scooped out

fresh thyme leaves, chopped

Add the onion, celery, chilli and garlic to a food processor and blitz until they are finely chopped.

Place a large saucepan over a high heat. Add the oil to the pan, followed by the blitzed onion mixture, then the paprika, thyme and bay. Sauté the mixture for 2–3 minutes, stirring often.

Turn the heat down to medium, then add the flour. Cook out the flour for a minute or so, then add the cream and stock. Mix well to remove any lumps.

Add the blitzed corn and allow the soup to come to a boil and thicken up for around 4–5 minutes.

Just before serving, cut the kernels off the charred corn cobs, and add to the soup with the soy sauce or tamari, seasoning and vegan cheese.

Serve the soup inside your bread bowl, and garnish with fresh chopped thyme leaves.

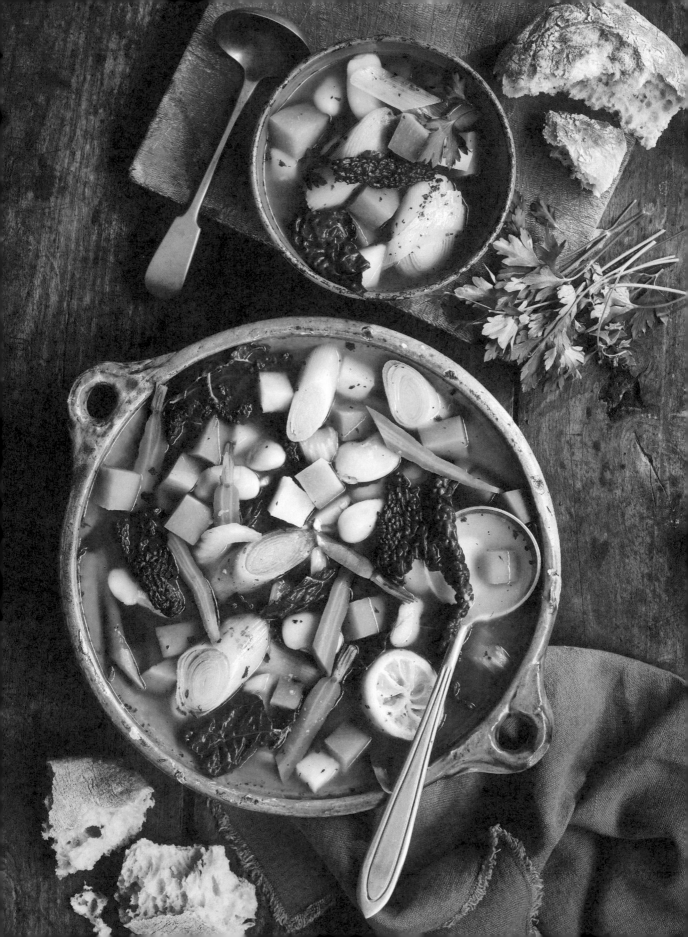

HEARTY WELSH CAWL

A dish from my home country, Wales. Usually made with lamb, this vegan version is just as bold and flavoursome, thanks to a few special umami-packed ingredients. It is just so warming and nourishing.

SERVES **4**	COOKS IN **65 MINS**	DIFFICULTY **3/10**

2 leeks

3 celery sticks

2 garlic cloves, minced

1 swede (rutabaga)

2 medium potatoes

2 carrots

1 tbsp olive oil

1 tsp sea salt

2 tsp cracked black pepper

3 litres (6 pints) vegetable stock

1 tbsp mint sauce

1 tbsp Marmite or miso paste

1 x 400-g (14-oz) can butter (lima) beans, drained and rinsed

large handful of cavolo nero or curly kale, stems removed and cut into bite-sized pieces

handful of flat-leaf parsley

juice of 1 lemon

Peel and chop all the vegetables into approximately 2cm (¾in) pieces. I like to slice the leek, carrot and celery at an angle, for presentation purposes.

Place a large saucepan over a low heat and add the oil. When it is hot, add the leek, celery and garlic then sauté for 2–3 minutes before adding the remaining vegetables and the seasoning.

Continue to sauté the vegetables for 5 minutes, getting a little colour on them, then deglaze the pan with the vegetable stock, mint sauce and Marmite.

Bring the soup to a simmer and let it bubble away until the swede is tender. This usually takes 25–30 minutes.

Once the swede (rutabaga) has cooked, add the butter (lima) beans, cavolo nero, parsley and lemon juice and stir. Add the lemon halves to the pan for extra flavour, if you like. Let the soup simmer for an additional 5 minutes before serving.

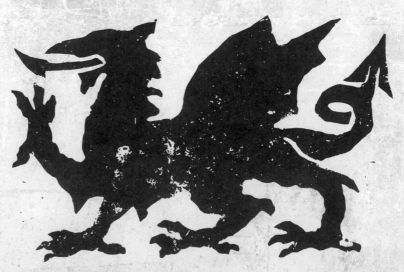

CREAMY MUSHROOM SOUP

| SERVES 4 | COOKS IN **60 MINS** | DIFFICULTY **3/10** | GF |

1 tbsp olive oil

2 onions, sliced

4 garlic cloves, minced

1 tbsp dried tarragon

1 tbsp dried thyme

1 tsp sea salt

2 tsp cracked black pepper

1kg (2lb 4oz) mixed mushrooms

240ml (1 cup) vegan-friendly white wine

1 litre (1¾ pints) hot vegetable stock

1 bay leaf

240ml (1 cup) vegan soy or oat cream, or coconut milk, plus a little extra for garnish

juice of ½ lemon

to garnish

fresh herbs, such as tarragon, parsley or thyme, chopped

1 tbsp truffle oil

Place a large saucepan over a low heat then add the oil. When hot, add the onions, garlic, dried herbs and seasoning. Sauté the mixture for 4–5 minutes, stirring often. You want to get the onions lovely and golden.

Next add about 90 per cent of the mushrooms to the pan. Reserve some to sauté later on for a garnish.

Turn up the heat to high and sauté the mushrooms for at least 10 minutes, stirring regularly. It may look like too many mushrooms at first but by the time you've finished sautéing them they will have shrunk down a lot.

After sautéing the mushrooms, deglaze the pan by adding the wine. Let it bubble away for a couple of minutes before adding the vegetable stock and bay leaf.

Bring the soup to a simmer before stirring in the vegan cream and lemon juice.

Let the soup bubble away for 20 minutes, stirring every now and then.

Before serving, blitz the soup in your blender until it's smooth and taste for seasoning, adjusting if necessary.

Sauté the reserved mushrooms in a little oil for a couple of minutes until golden, and top each bowl of soup with a few of mushrooms, some chopped fresh herbs and a drizzle of truffle oil.

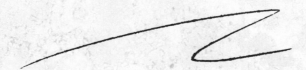

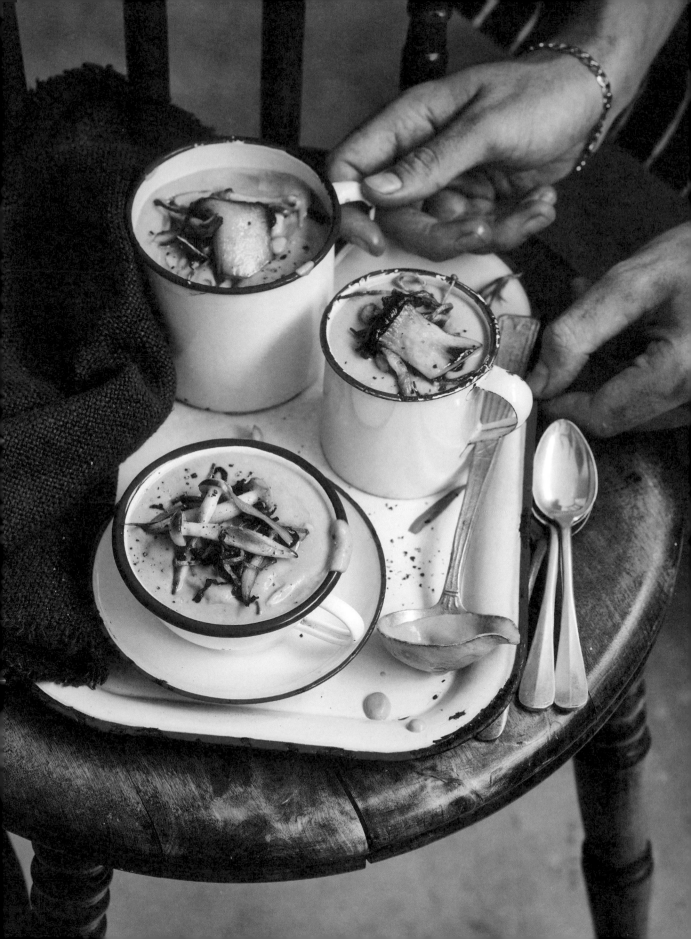

CAJUN PUMPKIN SOUP

SERVES **4**	COOKS IN **80 MINS**	DIFFICULTY **3/10**

(GF)

1 medium-sized pumpkin, peeled, deseeded and cubed (my pumpkin was 8kg/17lb 10oz)

3 tbsp Cajun spice mix

1 tbsp dried sage

drizzle of olive oil

2 onions, roughly chopped

3 garlic cloves, roughly chopped

480ml (2 cups) non-dairy milk

approx. 720ml (3 cups) hot vegetable stock (you may need more if your pumpkin is large)

squeeze of lemon juice, optional

sea salt and ground pepper

to garnish

handful of pumpkin seeds

drizzle of vegan cream, such as soy or oat

sprinkle of dried chilli flakes

toasted bread

Preheat your oven to 180°C (350°F).

Place the pumpkin into a roasting pan with the Cajun spice mix, sage, 2 teaspoons of salt and 1 teaspoon of pepper and a drizzle of oil. Mix it all up using your hands so the pumpkin is well coated.

Roast the pumpkin in your oven for around 45 minutes to 1 hour – or until it is tender.

When the pumpkin is cooked, place a large saucepan over a medium heat and add a drop of oil (or water if you're keeping this recipe oil-free). Add the chopped onion and garlic and sauté the mix with a pinch of salt for 4 minutes.

Add the roasted pumpkin to the saucepan, followed by the milk and vegetable stock.

Allow the soup to simmer for 10 minutes before blending it until super smooth. Blend the soup a few ladlefuls at a time and if it's too thick add more vegetable stock.

Check the soup is seasoned to your liking. If it needs an extra lift, add a squeeze of lemon juice, before serving with a few pumpkin seeds, a drizzle of vegan cream, a sprinkle of chilli flakes and some toasted bread.

This soup can be kept in the fridge for up to 4 days.

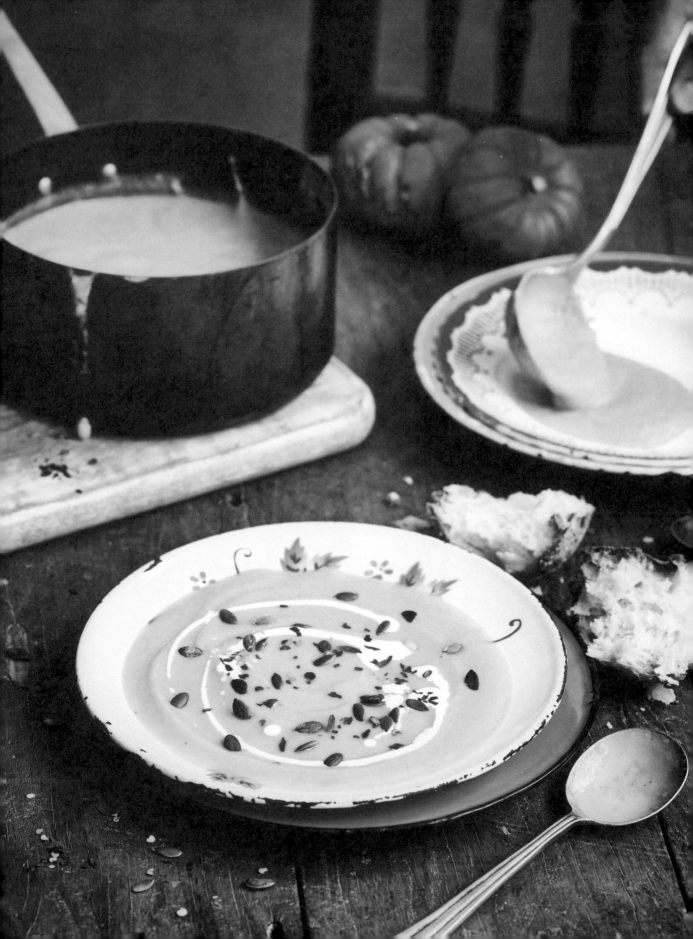

03

Light Bites

PEANUT-CRUSTED TOFU BITES

Jazz up your tofu by encrusting it in miso and peanuts. The fillets can be served with a dipping sauce as a snack or as part of a meal. They go great with rice or noodles. Make sure you use an extra-firm tofu for real meatiness.

SERVES **4**	COOKS IN **60 MINS**	DIFFICULTY **5/10**

2 x 280-g (10-oz) blocks of extra-firm tofu

2 tbsp smooth peanut butter

2 tbsp soy sauce or tamari

juice of 1 lime

pinch dried chilli flakes

½ tsp dried garlic

75g (¾ cup) shelled roasted peanuts, blitzed to a crumb

serve with

side salad

dipping sauce of your choice

First up, drain and pat dry the tofu using kitchen paper. Cut the blocks into slices.

Mix together the peanut butter, soy sauce or tamari, lime juice, chilli flakes and dried garlic.

Using a pastry brush, brush the peanut butter mix over each piece of tofu. If your mix isn't brushable, add a couple of tablespoons of water. Once the tofu blocks are coated, individually dip each piece into the peanut crumb and make sure they are nicely coated.

Once you've coated all of the tofu, place the pieces onto a baking sheet lined with greaseproof paper. Place the tray into your freezer for 20 minutes and preheat your oven to 180°C (350°F).

Remove the tofu from the freezer. Place a dry non-stick frying pan (skillet) over a medium heat and, when hot, lightly colour the coated tofu for around 2 minutes on each side.

Once golden, place the tofu back onto the baking sheet and then into your preheated oven for 15 minutes.

Serve your peanut-crusted tofu with a side salad and dipping sauce of your choice. I like to use Sriracha.

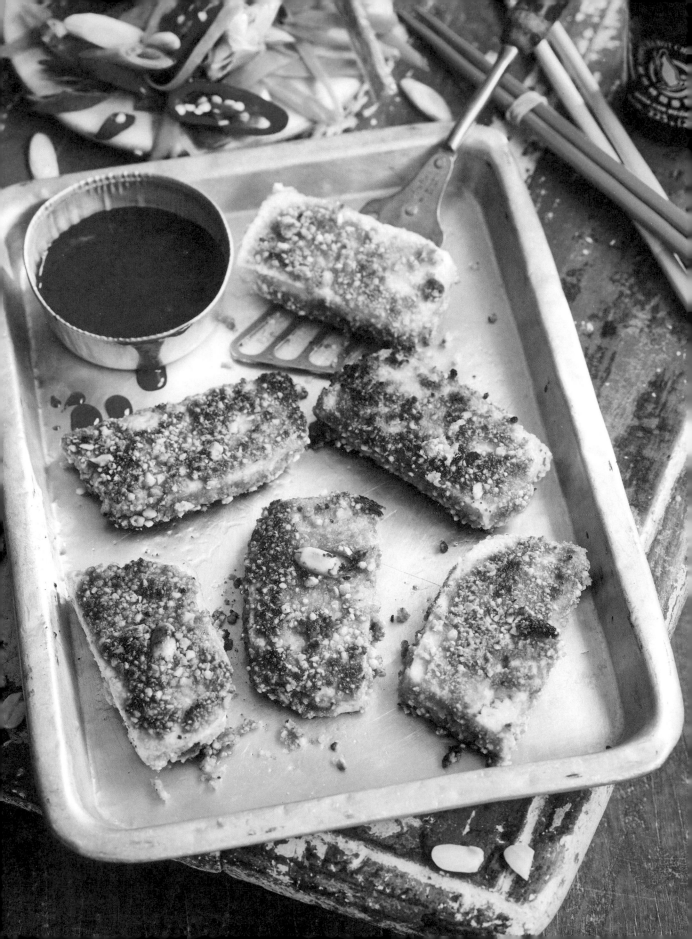

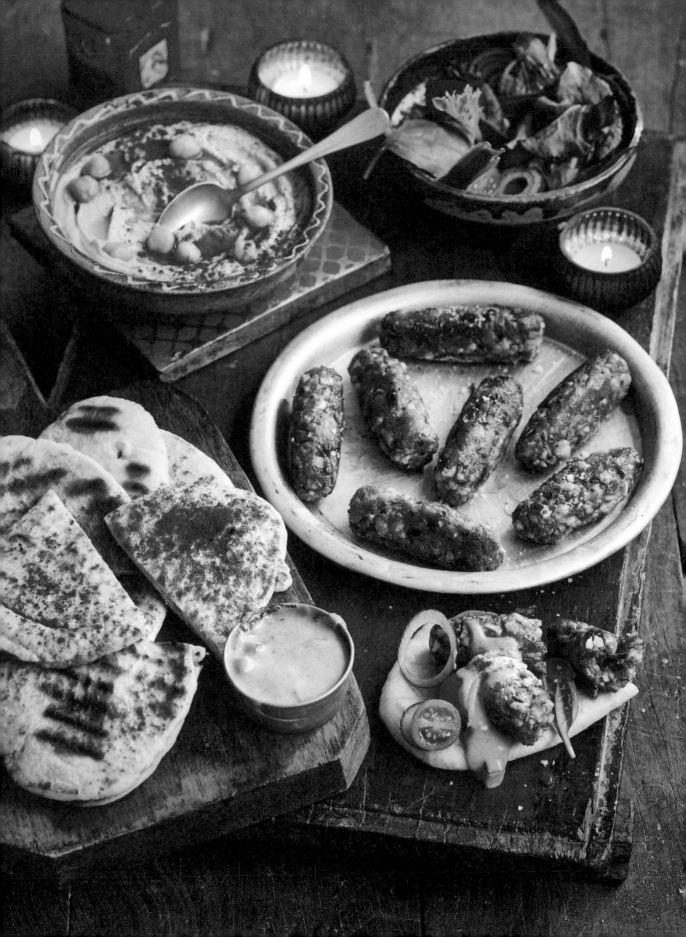

TOFU KOFTAS

| SERVES **4** | COOKS IN **30 MINS** | DIFFICULTY **5/10** |

for the koftas

1 x 280-g (10-oz) block of extra-firm tofu, pressed to remove excess water

3 spring onions (scallions), very finely sliced

3 garlic cloves, crushed

1 small red chilli, finely chopped

handful of mint, chopped

1 tsp ground cumin

1 tsp sweet smoked paprika

4 tbsp plain (all-purpose) flour

1 tbsp tomato purée

1 tsp sea salt

coconut oil, for frying

for the mint dip

245g (1 cup) vegan yogurt

¼ cucumber, de-seeded and finely chopped

1 tsp paprika

juice of ½ lemon

handful of fresh mint, chopped

serve with

warm pitta bread

simple salad of tomato, red onion, cucumber and lettuce leaves

hummus

Preheat your oven to 180°C (350°F) and line a baking sheet with greaseproof paper.

First up, make the koftas. Mash the tofu with an old-fashioned potato masher in a large mixing bowl, until it's broken up into small pieces. Add all the other kofta ingredients, apart from the coconut oil, to the bowl and mix using your hands until it comes together. If your mix is too wet, add a little more flour.

Take a couple of tablespoons of the mixture and form into a kofta shape with your hands. Repeat until you've used up all the mixture. Place the koftas onto the lined baking sheet.

Heat a non-stick frying pan (skillet) over a low heat, add the coconut oil and sauté the koftas in small batches, until golden. This should take approximately 3 minutes per batch. Place them back onto the tray, then when they are all done, put them into the oven to cook through for 15 minutes.

While the koftas are in the oven, mix together the mint dip ingredients in a small bowl.

Once the koftas are cooked, serve in warm pitta breads with salad, dip and hummus.

YAKITORI

These mushrooms are actually really MEATY and almost chicken-like when cooked. This is another dish that would be equally as good as a side dish. Leftover glaze can be stored in a sealed container for a few weeks.

MAKES **16**	COOKS IN **35 MINS**	DIFFICULTY **5/10**

CAN BE GF

for the glaze

240ml (1 cup) low-salt soy sauce or tamari

120ml (½ cup) water

200g (½ cup) sugar

3 tbsp rice vinegar

juice of ½ lime

½ tsp ground ginger

½ tsp garlic powder

½ tsp dried chilli flakes

2 tbsp cornflour (cornstarch), mixed with a little water

for the skewers

8 king oyster mushrooms

8 spring onions (scallions)

vegetable oil, for cooking

to serve

cooked rice (optional)

sprinkle of sesame seeds

chopped fresh chilli

Put all the glaze ingredients (except the cornflour/cornstarch) in to a saucepan and place over a medium heat. Bring the liquid to a simmer.

Allow to simmer for about 8 minutes before whisking in the cornflour mixture. The liquid should thicken up into a lovely glaze-like consistency. If it becomes too thick, add some water, and if too thin, slightly more cornflour/water mix, or just allow it to reduce down. Once thickened, remove it from the heat and set aside.

Cut the mushrooms in half lengthways, then cut each half into three, widthways. Cut the spring onions (scallions) to a similar size. Then skewer them up, alternating between mushrooms and spring onions.

Place a griddle pan over a high heat with a touch of oil (or get your barbecue nice and hot). Griddle each skewer for 4–5 minutes on each side, brushing over the glaze as they are cooking. Serve with a sprinkle of sesame seeds and fresh chilli.

Any leftover glaze is great to use as a sauce for stir fries.

Pictured on page 50.

CRISPY KICKIN' CAULIFLOWER

Cauliflower never tasted so good! These cauliflower bites really hit the spot – crispy, sticky, spicy and sweet. To keep the recipe oil free, bake them rather than frying.

SERVES **4**	COOKS IN **15 MINS**	DIFFICULTY **5/10**

CAN BE GF

500ml (2 cups) vegetable oil, for frying

1 head cauliflower, cut into small florets

sesame seeds, to serve

for the sauce

240ml (1 cup) orange juice

1 tbsp tomato purée

60ml (¼ cup) Sriracha sauce

1 tbsp soy sauce or tamari

2 tbsp maple syrup

1 tsp garlic powder

for the batter

100g (1 cup) cornflour (cornstarch)

240ml (1 cup) non-dairy milk

3 tbsp malt or rice vinegar

1 tsp sea salt

1 tsp baking powder

Put all the sauce ingredients into a small saucepan and mix well. Place the pan over a low heat and cook for 6 minutes to reduce down and thicken up, stirring occasionally.

To make the crispy cauliflower, place the vegetable oil in a large saucepan over a medium heat, making sure the oil reaches no more than halfway up the side of the pan. Alternatively, use a deep-fat fryer set to around 180°C (350°F).

Add the batter ingredients to a bowl and whisk together until smooth.

If using a saucepan, check the oil is hot enough by dipping a wooden spoon in; if bubbles form around it then your oil is ready.

Individually dip the cauliflower florets into the batter, then carefully lower them into the oil, a few at a time, cooking each one for around 2–3 minutes or until golden.

Once fried, remove the cauliflower florets from the oil with a slotted spoon and place each one onto a plate lined with kitchen paper to drain away any excess oil.

Toss the fried cauliflower in the thickened sauce, then sprinkle over the sesame seeds.

Pictured on page 51.

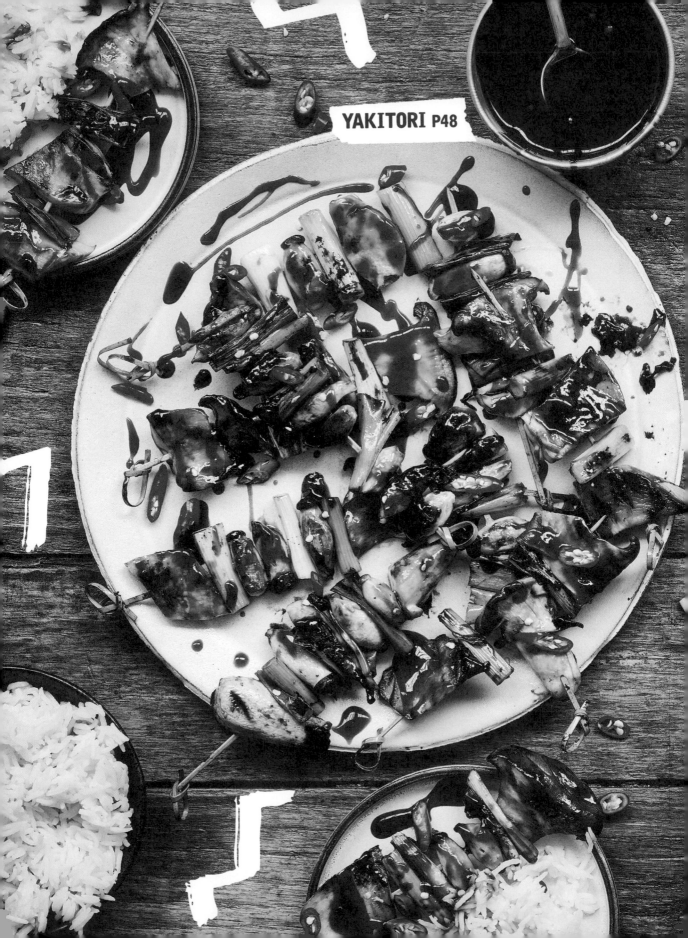

YAKITORI P48

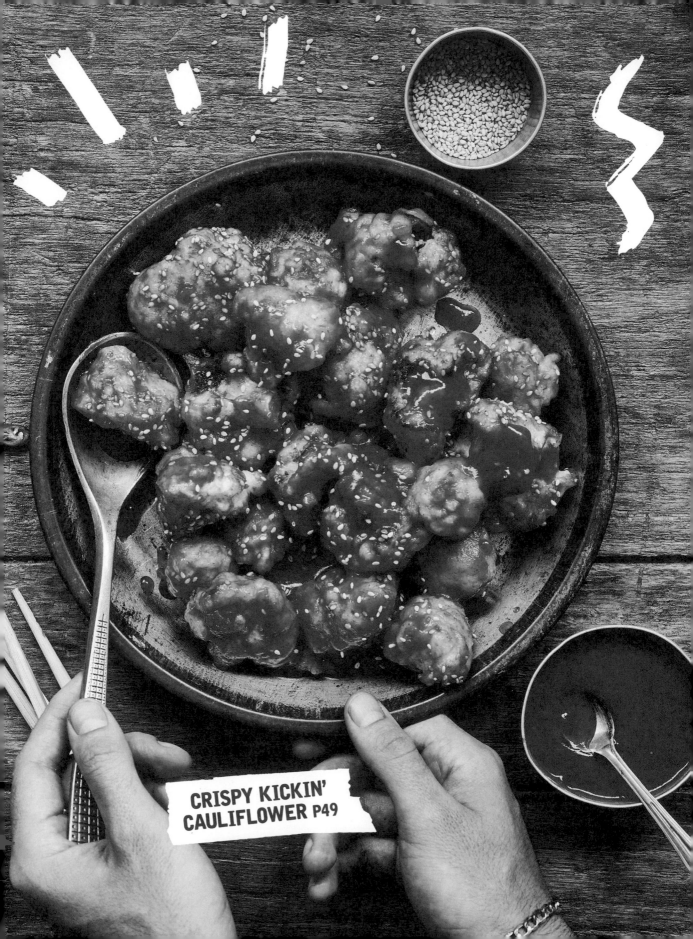

CRISPY KICKIN' CAULIFLOWER P49

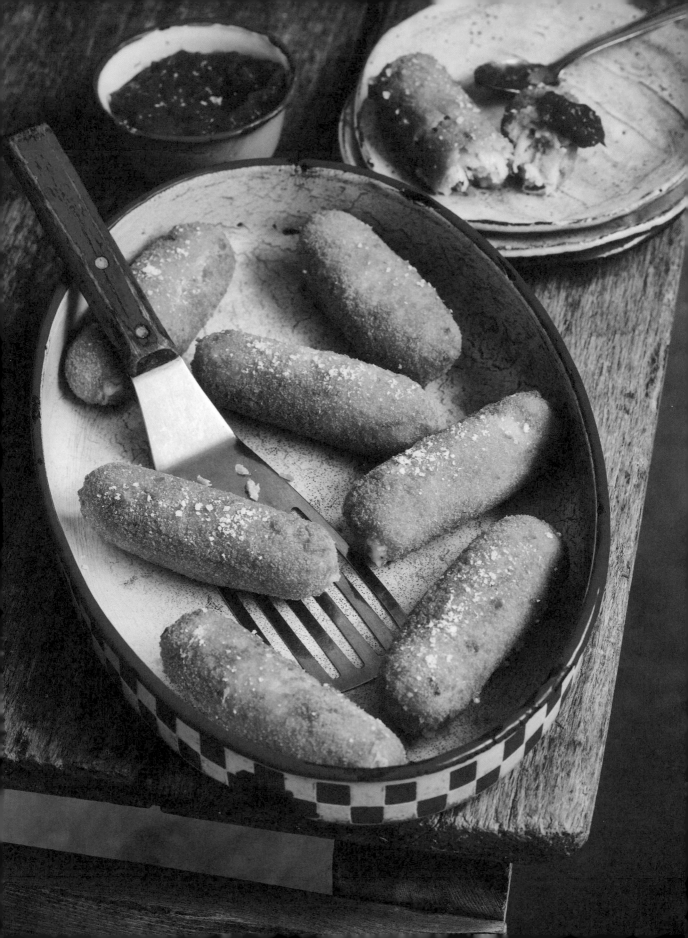

GLAMORGAN SAUSAGES

This is another classic dish from my home country, Wales. These sausages are a little more like croquettes, but I love anything coated in breadcrumbs, so these are the BEST!

MAKES **8**	COOKS IN **75 MINS**	DIFFICULTY **5/10**

2 tbsp vegetable oil, plus extra for drizzling

1 large leek, finely chopped

1 garlic clove, minced

handful of fresh sage, finely chopped

380g (2 cups) mashed potato

1 tbsp mustard

50g (½ cup) vegan cheese, grated

1 tbsp white miso paste

110g (1 cup) breadcrumbs

pinch sea salt and black pepper

for the coating

130g (1 cup) plain (all-purpose) flour or gluten-free flour

130g (1 cup) chickpea (gram) flour mixed with 240ml (1 cup) water

100g (2 cups) panko breadcrumbs

serve with

relish of your choice

Preheat your oven to 180°C (350°F) and line a baking sheet with greaseproof paper.

Heat the oil in a large frying pan (skillet) over a medium heat, add the leek and the garlic and sage, and sweat until soft. Set aside to cool.

Add the potato, mustard, cheese and miso to a mixing bowl and stir well. Add the cooled leek and the breadcrumbs, and mix with your hands until it all comes together.

Portion the mixture into 8 equal-sized pieces, then form into sausages.

Place the plain (all-purpose) flour, the chickpea (gram) flour mix, and the breadcrumbs in three separate bowls. Coat the sausages first in the flour, then in the gram mixture and finally the breadcrumbs.

Once coated, place the sausages onto the lined baking sheet. Drizzle a little oil over the sausages then bake for 30 minutes or until golden.

Serve immediately with a relish of your choice.

FIVE SPICE MUSHROOM SPRING ROLLS

| MAKES **8–10** | COOKS IN **90 MINS** | DIFFICULTY **7/10** |

1 pack spring-roll wrappers

2 tbsp plain (all-purpose) flour, mixed with enough water to make a paste-like consistency

1 litre (4 cups) vegetable oil, for frying

for the filling

2 tbsp vegetable oil

2 x 170-g (6-oz) punnets of mixed Asian mushrooms, such as enoki or oyster, cut into thin strips

sea salt

3 tsp Chinese five spice

2 carrots, peeled and julienned

1 red onion, finely sliced

¼ small white cabbage, outer leaves removed, finely shredded

handful of fresh beansprouts

2 tbsp soy sauce

1 tbsp hoisin sauce

3 tbsp rice wine vinegar

1 tbsp cornflour (cornstarch) mixed with 2 tbsp water

to serve

chopped spring onions (scallions)

black sesame seeds

soy sauce

dipping sauce of choice

First, make the filling. Place a wok over a high heat and add a touch of the oil. When hot, add the mushrooms and stir-fry for around 5–6 minutes. When the mushrooms have coloured and shrunk considerably, turn the heat down, then season with sea salt and the Chinese five spice. Cook for a minute or so to let the spices roast. Remove the mushrooms to a bowl and set aside.

Give the wok a wipe clean with kitchen paper, then add a touch more oil and place the pan back over a high heat. Add the carrots, red onion, cabbage and beansprouts and stir-fry for 3 minutes. Add the mushrooms back into the wok with the soy sauce, hoisin sauce and vinegar. Turn the heat down to low and allow the mixture to cook away for a couple of minutes. Stir in the cornflour (cornstarch) paste, then turn off the heat. Allow to cool to room temperature.

To form the spring rolls, start by laying one spring-roll wrapper on your work surface. Using a pastry brush, brush the flour mixture around the edge of the wrapper to form a border about 2cm (¾in) wide.

Neatly place around 3 tablespoons of the filling mixture on the wrapper in a diagonal strip from corner to corner, not going too close to the edges. Fold over the corners at each end of the strip of filling, then tightly roll up the spring roll, sealing at the top. Cover the spring roll right away with a damp kitchen cloth so it doesn't dry out. Repeat with the rest of the filling and wrappers. Once you've rolled all the mixture, you can either freeze the spring rolls and fry at a later date or fry right away.

Preheat your deep-fat fryer to 180°C (350°F) or use a large saucepan half-filled with oil over a medium heat. To test if the oil is hot enough for frying, place a wooden spoon into the oil. If bubbles form around it, it is hot enough.

Carefully lower 3–4 spring rolls into the oil and fry for around 4 minutes. Do not add too many as it will overcrowd the pan, lowering the temperature of the oil and raising the oil level, which can be very dangerous.

Once the spring rolls are golden and crispy, remove them from the oil using a spider or slotted spoon and place them onto a plate lined with kitchen paper. Serve with chopped spring onions (scallions), a sprinkle of sesame seeds, soy sauce and a dipping sauce of your choice.

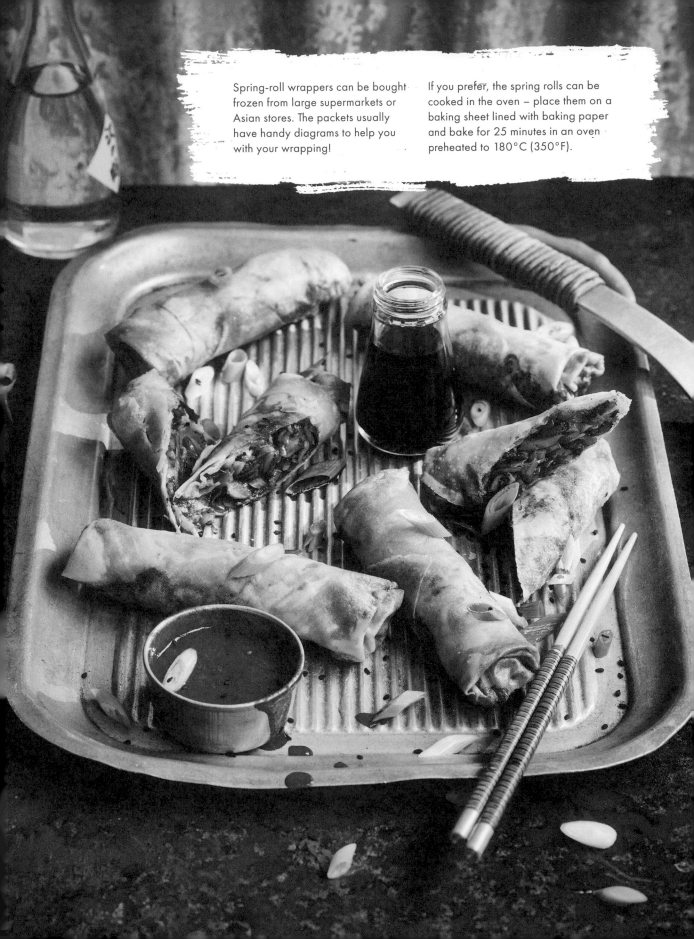

Spring-roll wrappers can be bought frozen from large supermarkets or Asian stores. The packets usually have handy diagrams to help you with your wrapping!

If you prefer, the spring rolls can be cooked in the oven – place them on a baking sheet lined with baking paper and bake for 25 minutes in an oven preheated to 180°C (350°F).

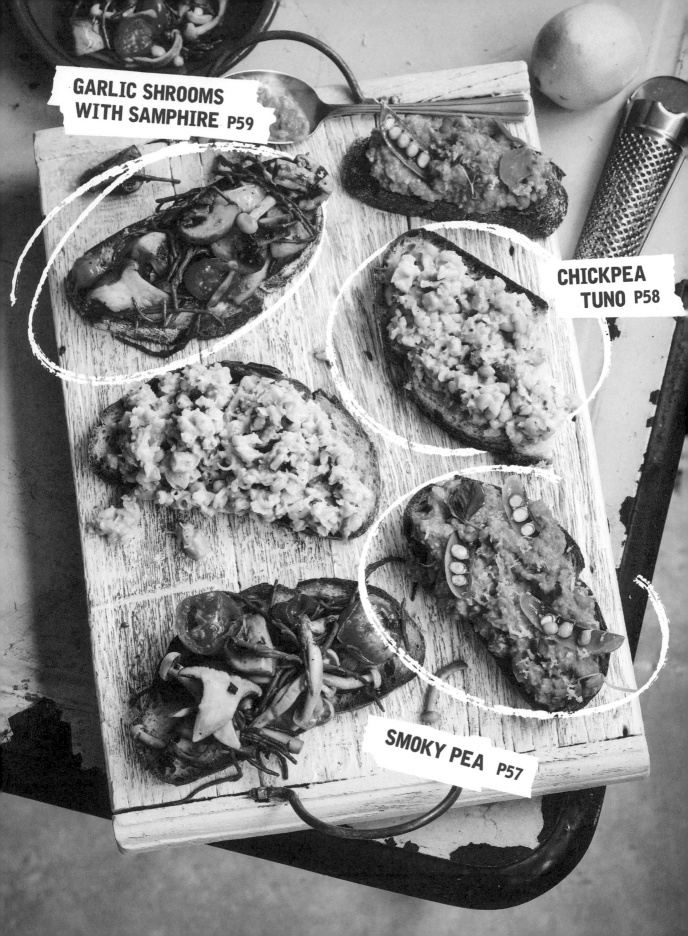

GARLIC SHROOMS
WITH SAMPHIRE P59

CHICKPEA
TUNO P58

SMOKY PEA P57

TOAST TOPPERS

Liven up your toast with these fantastic toppings. They also make great sandwich fillings. These recipes are a lifesaver for a speedy lunch. Serve them all together on a platter to impress your guests! You can even jazz up your toasted bread by pan-frying it in a little oil and garlic.

SMOKY PEA

SERVES **2**	COOKS IN **20 MINS**	DIFFICULTY **3/10**

drizzle of olive oil (or use water for oil-free cooking)

1 shallot, finely chopped

1 garlic clove, minced

½ tsp sweet smoked paprika

pinch each sea salt and black pepper

300g (2 cups) frozen peas

1 tbsp fresh mint leaves, chopped

240ml (1 cup) hot vegetable stock

2–3 drops liquid smoke (optional)

toasted bread, to serve

to garnish

juice and zest of 1 lemon

sugarsnap peas, halved

pea shoots

Heat the oil in a small non-stick saucepan over a very low heat. When hot, add the shallot, garlic, smoked paprika and seasoning.

Sauté for a couple of minutes before adding the peas and mint. Cook for 3–4 minutes before adding the stock and liquid smoke (if using). Bring to a simmer then remove from the heat and blitz the mixture in your blender (or use a stick blender). I only blend the peas lightly as I like them to have a nice crushed look.

Serve the peas on toasted bread with the garnishes.

CHICKPEA TUNO

| SERVES **4** | COOKS IN **15 MINS** | DIFFICULTY **3/10** |

15 MIN   PRO TEIN   GF

1 sheet nori seaweed

3 spring onions (scallions),
finely sliced

1 x 400-g (14-oz) can chickpeas
(garbanzos), drained and rinsed

1 tbsp malt vinegar

pinch sea salt

pinch cracked black pepper

4 tbsp vegan mayonnaise

150g (1 cup) sweetcorn

toasted bread

First, blitz the nori sheet in your blender until it's finely chopped.

Add of all the remaining ingredients, apart from the mayonnaise and the sweetcorn, to a mixing bowl.

Using a potato masher, mash the mix until the chickpeas (garbanzos) have been crushed.

Stir in the mayo and the sweetcorn, then add as little or as much of the chopped nori as you like. Just give it a taste and when it suits you, it's ready. Serve on toast.

Pictured on page 56.

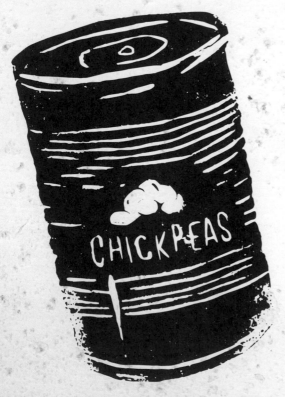

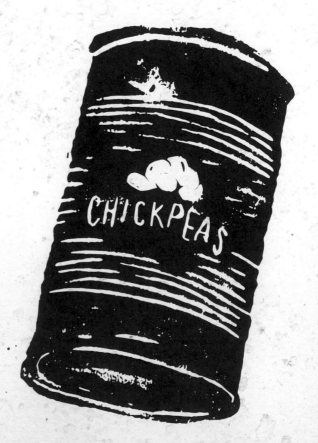

GARLIC SHROOMS WITH SAMPHIRE

| SERVES **2** | COOKS IN **15 MINS** | DIFFICULTY **3/10** |

15 MIN

1 tbsp olive oil

250g (9oz) closed cup mushrooms, halved

handful of cherry tomatoes, halved

1 tsp roasted garlic granules

pinch sea salt

pinch ground pepper

handful of samphire

handful of fresh parsley, chopped

vegan cream cheese

toasted bread

Heat the oil in a non-stick pan over a medium heat. Add the mushrooms, tomatoes, garlic, seasoning and samphire.

Sauté the mixture for 4–5 minutes, or until the mushrooms are lovely and golden.

Throw in the chopped parsley and toss the pan a couple of times.

Spread the cream cheese over the toast and serve the mushroom mixture on top.

Pictured on page 56.

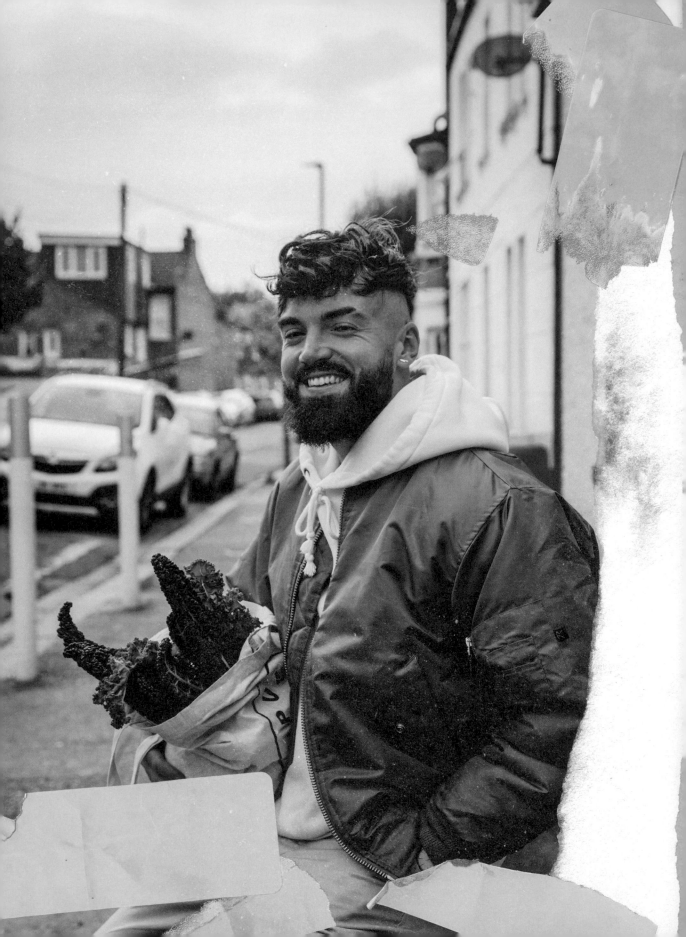

MUSHROOM 'PRAWN' TOASTS

I just had to try and veganize this hors d'oeuvre – a classic part of a
Chinese take-out. The nori adds a real taste of the sea.

SERVES **4**	COOKS IN **30 MINS**	DIFFICULTY **5/10**

4–5 tbsp sesame oil, for frying

1 shallot, finely chopped

2 x 170-g (6-oz) punnets of
mixed mushrooms

1 sheet nori, blitzed into
small pieces

juice of 1 lemon

120ml (½ cup) vegan-friendly
white wine

180ml (¾ cup) creamy
non-dairy milk

6 slices of white bread

280g (2 cups) mixed sesame seeds

sea salt and ground pepper

dipping sauce of choice, to serve

Heat a large frying pan (skillet) over a medium heat. Add a touch of sesame
oil then the shallot and mushrooms. Sauté for 5 minutes, stirring often.

Add seasoning, nori, lemon juice and white wine. Cook for a further
4 minutes.

Transfer the mushroom mixture to a blender, with the milk. Blitz until it
forms a paste-like consistency.

Preheat your oven to 180°C (350°F).

Spread the mushroom mix onto your slices of bread and generously sprinkle
sesame seeds over the top, pressing them on with your hands.

Heat a large non-stick pan over a low heat and add some sesame oil.
Carefully place a slice of bread into the pan and cook on each side for
3 minutes.

Once the toasts have been fried, place them onto a baking sheet then bake
in the oven for 12 minutes.

Serve the baked toasts with a dipping sauce of your choice, with each slice
cut into quarters.

Pictured on page 109.

MUSHROOM BUCKWHEAT CRÊPES WITH ASPARAGUS

| SERVES **2** | COOKS IN **15 MINS** | DIFFICULTY **5/10** |

90g (¾ cup) buckwheat flour

1 tsp baking powder

1 tsp sea salt

1 tsp black pepper

2 tbsp chopped fresh chives

240ml (1 cup) non-dairy milk

4 tbsp vegetable oil, for frying

for the mushroom filling

1 x 170g (6oz) punnet mixed mushrooms, chopped

6 asparagus spears, woody part removed and cut into 3 pieces

2 tsp garlic granules

1 tsp dried chilli

1 tbsp dried tarragon

35ml (1 shot) vegan-friendly brandy

240ml (1 cup) vegan cream

2 tsp sea salt

1 tsp cracked black pepper

to serve

mixed seeds

salad leaves

zest of 1 lemon

First up, get the crêpes going. To a mixing bowl, add the flour, baking powder, salt, pepper and chives, then mix well.

Pour in the non-dairy milk and whisk everything together until it's a smooth thin pancake-batter consistency.

Preheat a large non-stick frying pan (skillet) over a medium heat and add a touch of vegetable oil. When hot, ladle in enough batter to cover the base of the pan. I use the back of my ladle to spread the batter out.

Cook the crêpe for around 2 minutes on each side, using a palette knife to help flip it over. Repeat the process until you've used up all the batter, adding more oil to the pan as needed.

While the crêpes are cooking, preheat another non-stick pan over a high heat. Add a touch of oil, followed by the mushrooms, asparagus, garlic, chilli and tarragon. Sauté for 3–4 minutes, stirring often. When the mushrooms are golden, deglaze pan with the brandy. You may see a few flames when you add it – that's just the alcohol burning off – exciting, but please be careful!

A minute after adding the brandy, add the vegan cream and seasoning. Let the creamy mixture come to a simmer for 1 minute, then serve up.

Fill your crêpes with plenty of the mushroom mixture, some salad leaves and a sprinkle of mixed seeds. Grate over some lemon zest, to finish.

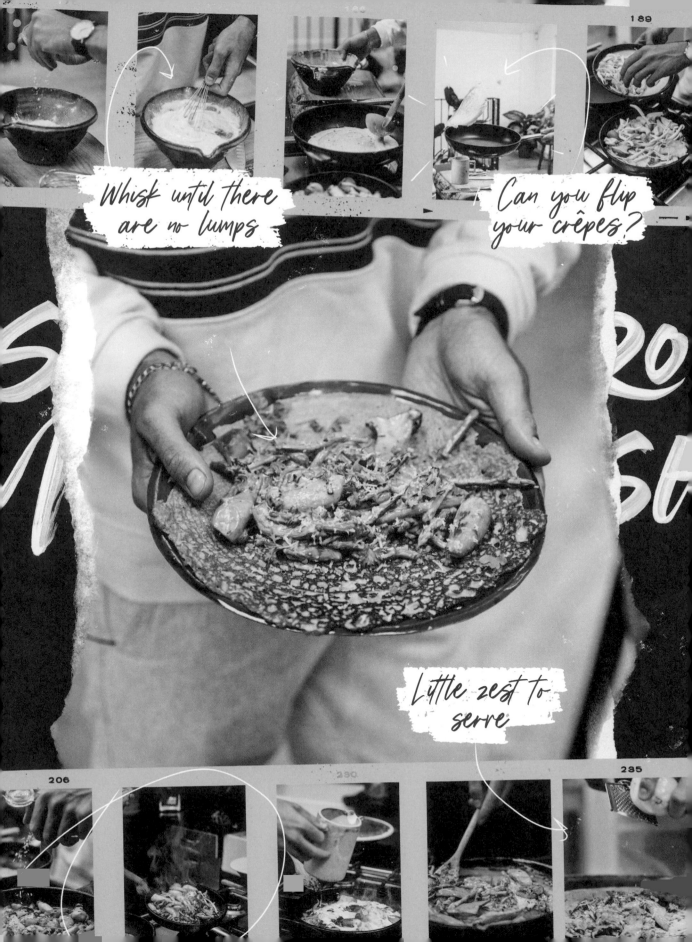

Whisk until there are no lumps

Can you flip your crêpes?

Little zest to serve

04

PERFECT PASTA

Perfect Pasta

MY FAMOUS LASAGNE

| SERVES **6** | COOKS IN **90 MINS** | DIFFICULTY **5/10** |

for the béchamel sauce

900ml (4 cups) soy or oat milk

1 onion

1 bay leaf

pinch nutmeg

1 tsp sea salt

1 tsp white pepper

115g (½ cup) vegan margarine

70g (½ cup) plain (all-purpose) flour or gluen-free flour

100g (1 cup) grated vegan cheese and/or 2 tbsp nutritional yeast (optional)

for the ragu

2 tbsp olive oil

1 red onion, finely sliced

3 garlic cloves, minced

4 celery sticks, finely sliced

3 tbsp tomato purée

1 courgette (zucchini), diced

1 aubergine (eggplant), diced

1 tbsp mixed herbs

650g (4 cups) vegan mince

2 tbsp balsamic vinegar

2 x 400-g (14-oz) cans chopped tomatoes

pinch sea salt

1 pack lasagne sheets

fresh basil, to serve

First up, infuse the milk for the béchamel. Add the soy or oat milk to a medium saucepan, followed by the onion, bay, nutmeg and seasonings. Place the saucepan over a low heat and cook, stirring every now and then, allowing hthe flavours to infuse for 15 minutes.

To make the ragu, place a large saucepan over a medium heat. Add the oil, followed by the onion, garlic, celery, tomato purée and a pinch of salt. Sweat the mix down for around 3–4 minutes.

Add the courgette (zucchini), aubergine (eggplant) and mixed herbs. Turn the heat down to low, pop a lid on the pan and cook for 3–4 minutes. Add the vegan mince and stir well. Cook for a further 2–3 minutes.

Deglaze the pan with the balsamic vinegar and chopped tomatoes, then pop the lid back on and cook over a low heat for 10–15 minutes.

To make the béchamel, add the vegan margarine to a large saucepan and place over a low heat. When the margarine is melted, add the flour. Mix well, using a spatula. Stir the mixture for a couple of minutes to cook out the flour.

Gradually whisk in the infused milk, a little at a time. Once you've added all the milk, the béchamel should be creamy. If you want to make it cheesy, whisk in the vegan cheese and/or nutritional yeast.

Meanwhile, preheat your oven to 180°C (350°F).

Build your lasagne in an ovenproof baking dish, a layer at a time. I like to do a layer of ragu, then béchamel, then pasta sheets. Repeat until you have filled your dish, ending with a layer of béchamel.

Bake the lasagne for 45 minutes. Serve with a few fresh basil leaves.

This works just as well using the same weight of chopped mushrooms or lentils in place of the vegan mince.

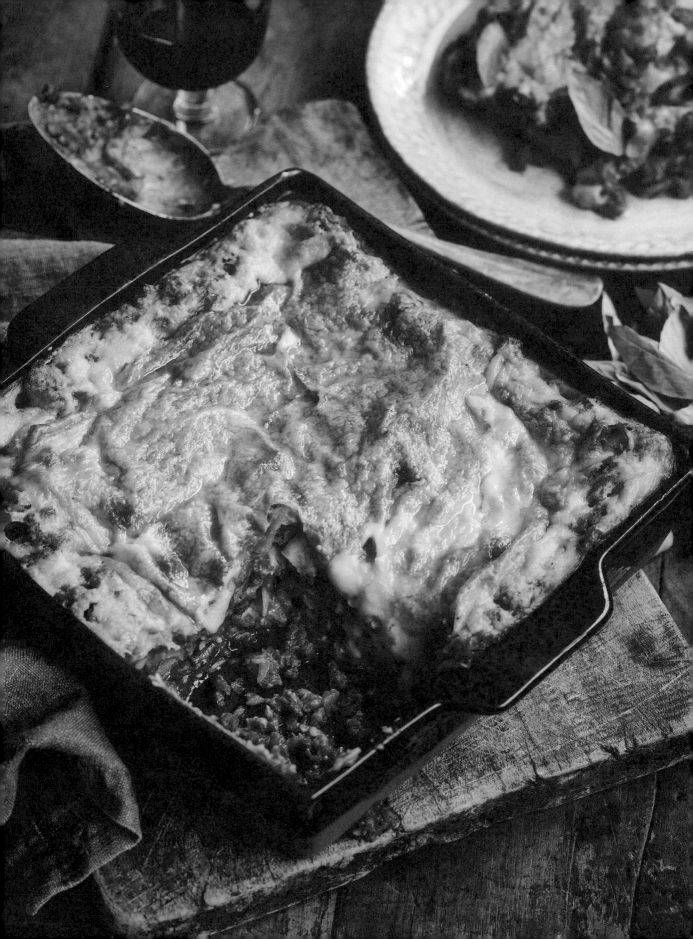

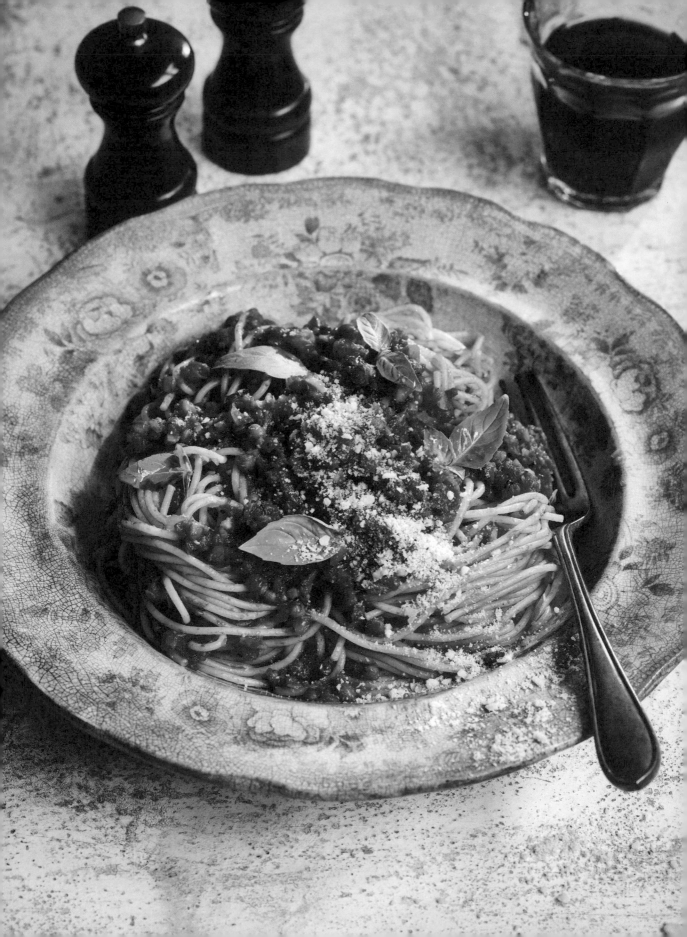

SIMPLE LENTIL SPAGHETTI BOLOGNESE

| SERVES **4** | COOKS IN **45 MINS** | DIFFICULTY **3/10** |

1 large onion, roughly chopped

2 celery sticks, roughly chopped

6 garlic cloves

1 carrot, roughly chopped

2 tbsp vegetable oil

1 tbsp dried mixed herbs

4 tbsp tomato purée

1 tsp sea salt

1 tsp cracked black pepper

1 tbsp miso paste

2 x 400g (14oz) cans chopped tomatoes

240ml (1 cup) vegan-friendly red wine

2 x 400-g (14-oz) cans cooked green lentils, drained

for the 'parmesan' topping

3 tbsp toasted flaked almonds

3 tbsp nutritional yeast

serve with

400g (14oz) spelt spaghetti or other egg-free pasta, cooked according to packet instructions

fresh basil leaves

Add the onion, celery, garlic and carrot to a blender and blitz until everything is finely chopped.

Place a large saucepan over a medium heat. Add the oil to the pan, followed by the blitzed vegetables. Sauté for 4–5 minutes or until softened, then add the mixed herbs, tomato purée and seasoning. Cook for a couple of minutes before adding the miso, chopped tomatoes and wine. Turn the heat down to low and place a lid on the pan. Allow the sauce to simmer away for 20 minutes.

Add the lentils, and cook for a further 5 minutes.

Meanwhile, to make the 'parmesan' topping, blitz together the toasted almonds with the nutritional yeast until the mixture resembles a fine crumb.

Serve the Bolognese with spaghetti, a sprinkle of the 'parmesan' topping and some fresh basil.

Generally, dried pasta is egg-free, so vegan-friendly, but be sure to check the packaging. Choosing wholewheat or spelt options will make a pasta dish more nutritious.

SUN-DRIED TOMATO & BROCCOLI PASTA

SERVES **4**	COOKS IN **15 MINS**	DIFFICULTY **3/10**

15 MIN **CAN BE GF**

300g (10½oz) dried pasta

2 tbsp olive oil

1 head of broccoli,
cut into small florets

3 tbsp flaked almonds

black pepper

handful of fresh basil, chopped,
plus extra to serve

squeeze of lemon juice

for the sauce

8–10 sun-dried tomatoes

1 tsp dried chilli flakes

4 garlic cloves

1 tbsp nutritional yeast (optional)

2 tbsp tomato purée

zest of ½ lemon

juice of 1 lemon

pinch sea salt

for the pangrattato

2 tbsp extra virgin olive oil

220g (2 cups) breadcrumbs

zest and juice of 1 lemon

1 tsp garlic powder

pinch sea salt

3 tsp dried mixed herbs

First up, get your pasta cooking in some salted boiling water, according to the packet instructions.

To make the sauce, rehydrate the sun-dried tomatoes by placing them in a small bowl with a ladleful of the pasta water for around 1 minute. Once they have slightly softened, add them to a blender with the rest of the sauce ingredients and a few tablespoons of the rehydrating water (reserve the rest of the water). Blitz the mixture to a smooth paste.

Heat a large saucepan over a medium heat, add a touch of oil, followed by the broccoli and flaked almonds. Sauté for a couple of minutes or until the almonds are golden. Add the sun-dried tomato sauce to the pan and stir well, making sure the broccoli is fully coated. Add the reserved rehydrating water from the tomatoes and a little extra pasta water to make it more saucy.

Let the sauce and broccoli cook away for 3–4 minutes over a low heat and stir every now and then.

Meanwhile, make the crispy breadcrumbs (aka pangrattato). Place a non-stick frying pan (skillet) over a low heat, add the oil, then add the breadcrumbs, lemon zest and juice, garlic, salt and herbs. Toast the breadcrumbs for a few minutes until they are nice and golden.

Once your pasta is cooked, drain and add the pasta to the sauce. Mix really well, making sure all the pasta is coated. Add some black pepper, the chopped fresh basil and a squeeze of lemon juice.

Serve your pasta with plenty of the pangrattato and a few fresh basil leaves.

If you are making this for someone with a nut allergy, use mixed seeds in place of the flaked almonds.

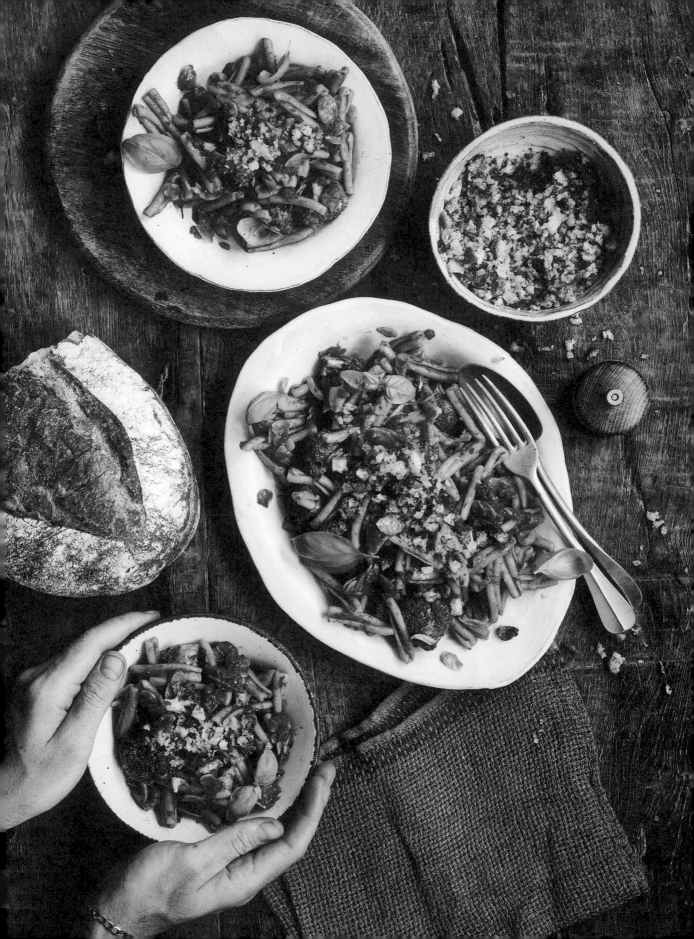

ZINGY FARFALLE

This is absolutely delicious – probably one of my favourite pasta dishes
I've ever made!

SERVES **2**	COOKS IN **15 MINS**	DIFFICULTY **3/10**

300g (10½oz) dried farfalle pasta

2 tbsp olive oil

1 white onion, sliced

1 red chilli

4 garlic cloves, sliced

2 large handfuls cavolo nero, shredded, stems removed

200g (7oz) broccolini, trimmed

1 fennel bulb, outer layer removed and discarded, finely sliced

120ml (½ cup) vegan-friendly white wine

zest and juice of 1 lemon, to serve

for the dressing

zest of 1 lemon, plus juice

2 tbsp capers

handful of fresh parsley

handful of fresh basil

handful of pine nuts

2 tsp sea salt

2 tsp black pepper

Get your pasta cooking in some salted boiling water, according to the packet instructions.

Meanwhile, heat a large non-stick pan over a medium heat and add the oil. Add the onion, chilli and garlic and sauté for a couple minutes.

Add the cavolo nero, the broccolini and the fennel and continue to gently sauté.

Meanwhile, add the dressing ingredients to a blender and blitz to a purée. Alternatively, grind everything together in a pestle and mortar. Add the dressing to the pan with the vegetables and sauté for a couple of minutes before deglazing the pan with the white wine and a ladleful of the pasta cooking water. Turn the heat down to low and let the sauce cook away for a couple of minutes.

Once your pasta is cooked, drain and add the pasta to the sauce. Toss and stir the pasta until it's coated in all the lovely flavours. Serve your pasta right away, with extra lemon juice and zest.

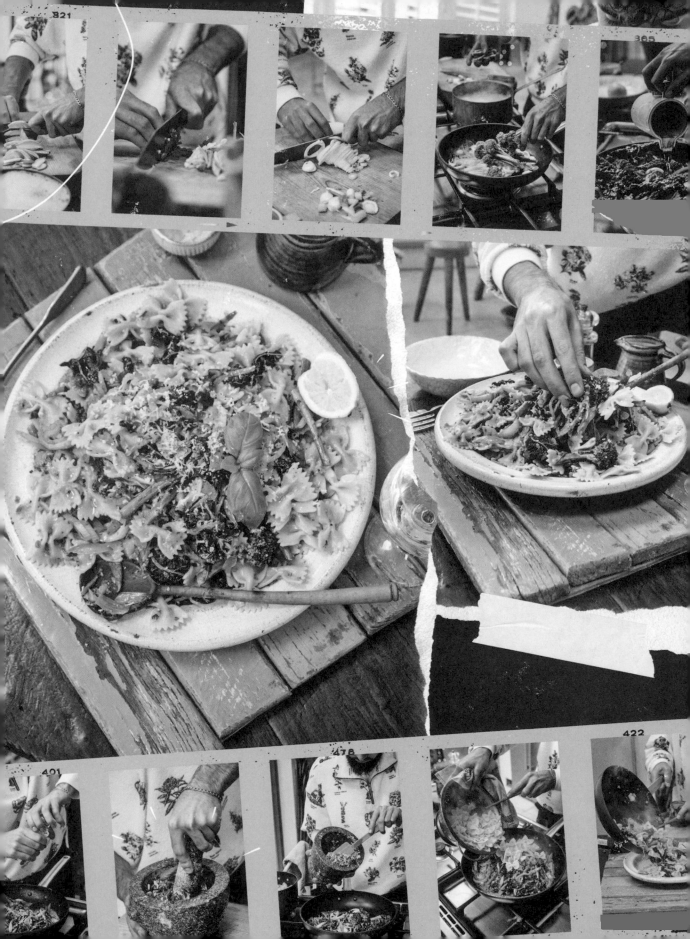

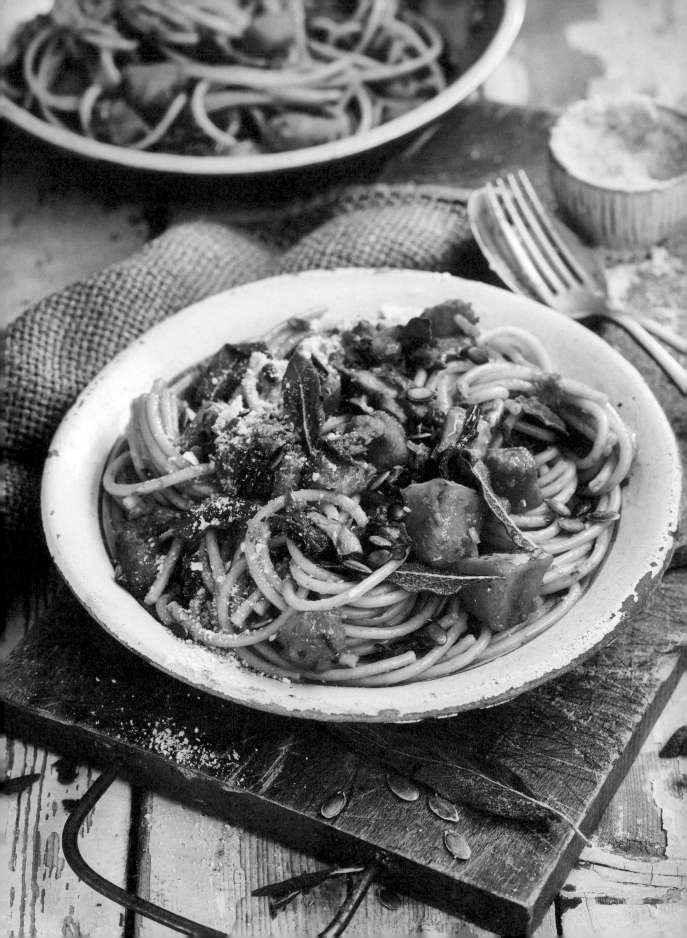

SUPER SQUASH, SAGE & SHIITAKE PASTA

SERVES 4	COOKS IN **90 MINS**	DIFFICULTY **5/10**

1 butternut squash, halved length-wise, seeds removed

2 tbsp olive oil

400g (14oz) wholewheat pasta

1 onion, roughly chopped

3 garlic cloves, peeled

1 small red chilli

4 sun-dried tomatoes

6 fresh sage leaves

8 shiitake mushrooms, finely sliced

1 tsp smoked paprika

2 tbsp balsamic vinegar

sea salt and cracked black pepper

to garnish

crispy sage leaves (optional)

4 tbsp pumpkin seeds

vegan cheese

Preheat your oven to 180°C (350°F).

Place the two halves of squash, cut side up onto a baking tray. Drizzle over a touch of oil and sprinkle over some seasoning then roast for about 55 minutes or until the squash is soft. Remove from the oven and allow to cool slightly.

Get your pasta cooking in a pan of salted boiling water according to the packet instructions.

Scoop out the cooled butternut squash flesh, and place it in a bowl.

Add the onion, garlic, chilli, sun-dried tomatoes and sage to a blender and blitz until finely chopped. Alternatively, just finely slice everything by hand (blitzing is just that little bit faster!).

Place a large non-stick saucepan over a medium heat. When the pan is hot, add a touch of olive oil, followed by the onion mixture. Sauté with a sprinkling of salt for 3–4 minutes. This is where the sauce will develop a great base flavour.

Add the shiitake mushroom, and cook for another 3–4 minutes, getting them really lovely and golden and crisp... there's nothing worse than soggy mushrooms!

Deglaze the pan with the balsamic vinegar, then add the squash flesh and 1 teaspoon of black pepper. Cook for 4 minutes, letting the flavours mingle and getting some lovely colour on the squash. Add a small ladleful of pasta cooking water to make it slightly more saucy, then add the cooked drained pasta. Mix everything together making sure your pasta is coated nicely.

To make crispy sage leaves for the garnish, simply fry them in a little olive oil for a couple of minutes until crispy.

To serve the pasta, sprinkle over some pumpkin seeds and add the crispy sage leaves to garnish. Top with some grated vegan cheese.

INCREDIBLE ONE-POT TOMATO PASTA

You might be surprised by how elegant this one-pot is. Your friends and family will never guess how simple this pasta dish is to prepare, I promise!

SERVES **2**	COOKS IN **25 MINS**	DIFFICULTY **3/10**

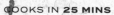

1 POT   CAN BE GF

200g (7oz) dried pasta

1 onion, finely sliced

1 garlic clove, minced

12 cherry tomatoes

2 tbsp tomato purée

handful of flat-leaf parsley, chopped

240ml (1 cup) vegan-friendly white wine

240ml (1 cup) vegetable stock

handful of pitted black olives, chopped

3 tbsp capers

pinch sea salt

2 tsp ground black pepper

Simply place all the ingredients into a large heavy-based saucepan and put a lid on.

Place the saucepan over a low heat and cook for 15–18 minutes. Stir every now and then. When the pasta is cooked, the dish is ready.

Pop the saucepan into the middle of your dinner table and dish up.

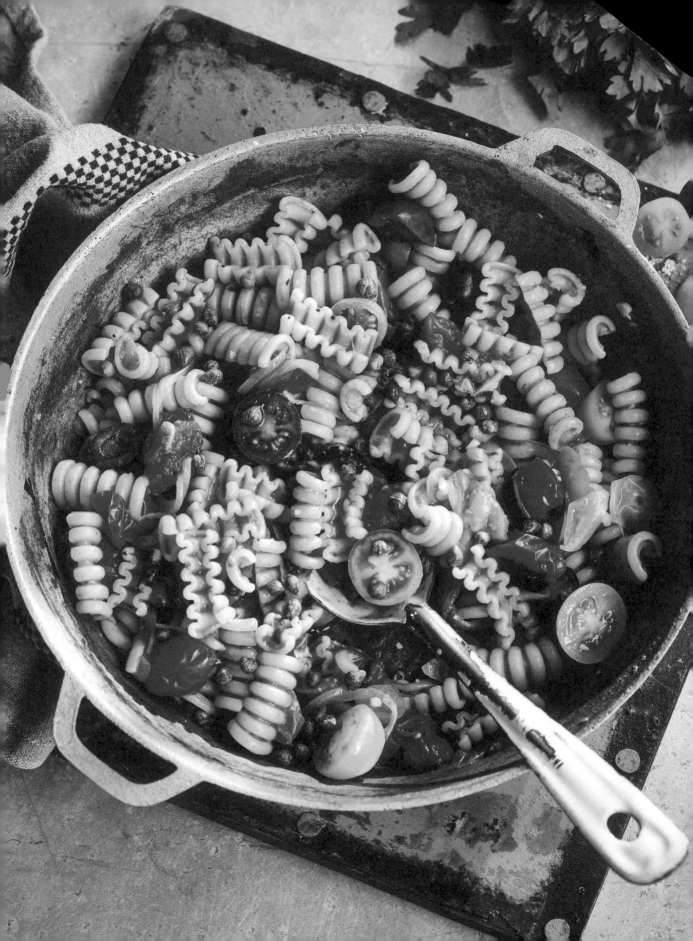

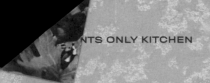
SPICY ARRABBIATA PASTA

| SERVES **4** | COOKS IN **40 MINS** | DIFFICULTY **3/10** |

CAN BE GF

15 cherry tomatoes, halved

1 red (bell) pepper, deseeded and finely sliced

3 tbsp olive oil

1 onion, finely chopped

6 garlic cloves, minced

1–2 red chillies (to taste), finely chopped

2 tsp sea salt

2 tsp cracked black pepper

2 x 400-g (14-oz) cans chopped tomatoes

2 tbsp caster (superfine) sugar

2 tbsp white wine vinegar

400g (14oz) dried pasta

handful of fresh basil, finely chopped, plus extra leaves to serve

Preheat your grill (broiler) to high. Line a baking sheet with foil and place the cherry tomatoes and red (bell) peppers on it, cut-side up, and drizzle with some of the oil.

Place the tray under the grill (broiler) for 10–12 minutes or until the tomatoes have gone a little crisp and golden. Set them aside. Cooking them in this way enhances the sweetness and all-round flavour.

Place a large non-stick saucepan over a medium heat and add a drizzle of oil followed by the onion, garlic, chilli and salt and pepper. Sauté for 2 minutes.

Add the chopped tomatoes, sugar and vinegar. Turn the heat down to low and let the sauce cook away for 12–15 minutes, stirring every now and then.

At this point, get your pasta cooking in salted boiling water, according to the packet instructions.

The sauce should now have thickened up considerably and reduced down, intensifying the flavour. Stir through the chopped basil, along with the grilled cherry tomatoes and (bell) peppers.

When the pasta has cooked, drain and mix it through the sauce, making sure it's well coated.

Serve up your pasta immediately, simply garnished with some fresh basil.

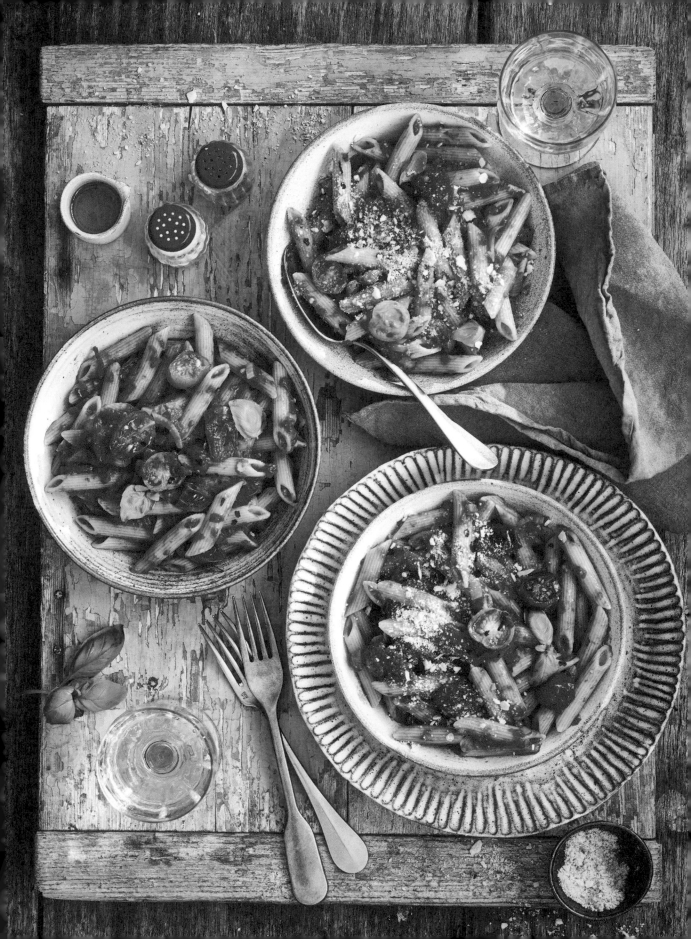

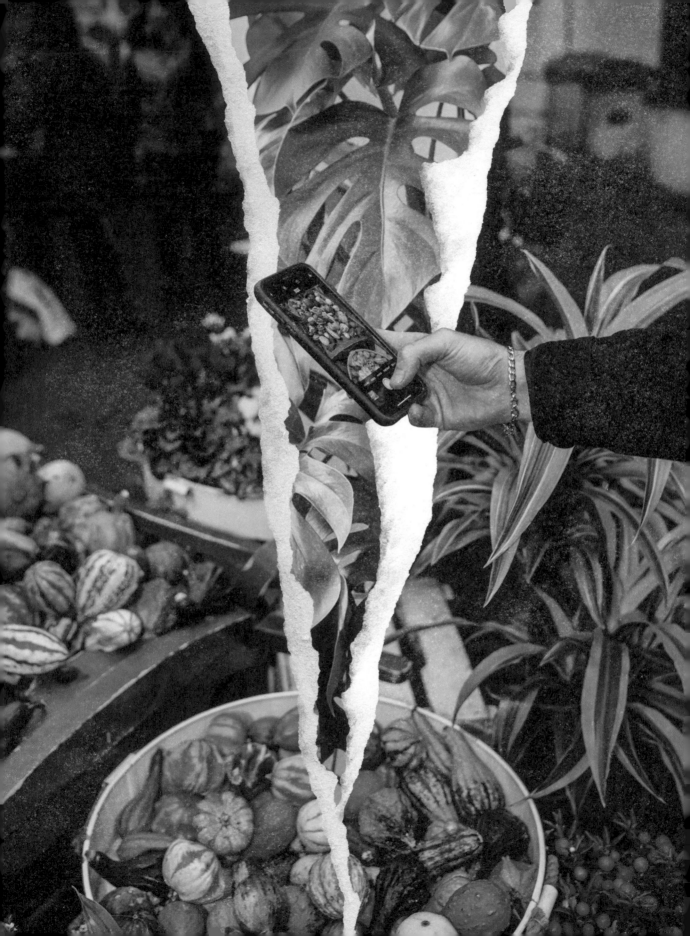

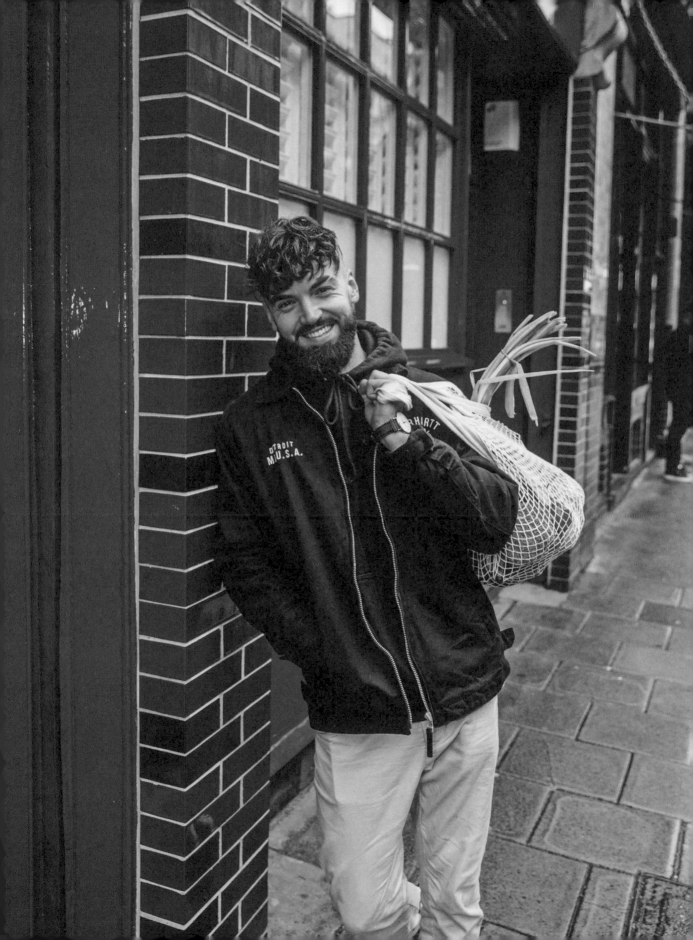

05

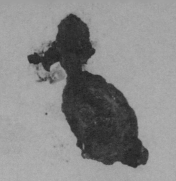

POW-ERFUL CURRIES

Powerful Curries

CHICKPEA CURRY WITH TURMERIC RICE

| SERVES **4** | COOKS IN **30 MINS** | DIFFICULTY **5/10** |

2 tbsp vegetable oil

1 onion, finely chopped

3 garlic cloves, minced

1 hot red chilli, finely chopped

thumb-sized piece of fresh ginger, peeled and minced

3 tsp sea salt

1 tsp ground turmeric

1 tsp mustard seeds

1 tsp ground coriander

1 tsp ground cumin

4 curry leaves

1 tsp ground fenugreek

2 tbsp tomato purée

2 x 400-g (14-oz) cans chickpeas (garbanzos), drained

1 x 400-ml (14-fl oz) can coconut milk

1 tbsp coconut flour

fresh coriander (cilantro), to serve

1 tbsp black onion seeds, to serve

for the rice

200g (1 cup) basmati rice, washed

½ tsp ground turmeric

1 cinnamon stick

1 cardamon pod

pinch sea salt

Place a large saucepan over a medium heat and add the oil. When hot, add the onion, garlic, chilli and ginger. Cook for 10 minutes, stirring often. This is the most important part of making the curry! Getting your base ingredients lovely and golden will ensure that the finished curry has a powerful flavour.

Add the salt and all the spices and cook, continuously stirring, for another 3–4 minutes. This will allow the spices to roast and release their aromatics. Throw in the tomato purée and cook for 1 more minute before adding the chickpeas (garbanzos). Stir well so they are coated in all the beautiful flavours.

Deglaze the pan with the coconut milk and stir once more, then allow it to come to a simmer. Let your curry bubble away gently for around 12 minutes.

Meanwhile, make the rice. Add the rice, turmeric, cinnamon stick, cardamon and salt to a small saucepan, along with 480ml (2 cups) water, pop the lid on and place the pan over a low heat to cook gently for around 12 minutes or until the liquid has been absorbed by the rice and it's perfectly cooked.

When the rice is cooked, and just before serving, stir the coconut flour into the curry to thicken it up a little.

Serve up your curry with the rice, a few fresh coriander (cilantro) leaves and a sprinkle of black onion seeds.

Pictured on page 86.

TRINIDADIAN DOUBLES

| SERVES **6** | COOKS IN **120 MINS** | DIFFICULTY **7/10** |

1 batch Chickpea Curry (opposite) – use a Scotch bonnet chilli and 1 tbsp Caribbean curry powder instead of all the spices

for the baras

2 tsp active dried yeast

195g (1½ cups) strong white bread flour

195g (1½ cups) plain (all-purpose) flour, plus extra for dusting

1 tsp sea salt

1 tsp ground turmeric

1 tsp ground cumin

2 tsp caster (superfine) sugar

1 tsp baking powder

2 tbsp olive oil, plus extra for greasing

1.5 litres (2½ pints) vegetable oil

for the tamarind sauce

115g (½ cup) tamarind paste

¼ Scotch bonnet chilli

1 onion

2 garlic cloves

juice of 1 lime

2 tsp fresh thyme leaves

3 tbsp caster (superfine) sugar

for the cucumber salsa

1 cucumber, seeds removed, grated

½ tsp sea salt

pinch dried chilli flakes

First, make the baras. Whisk the yeast with 315ml (1½ cups) lukewarm water in a measuring jug, then set aside for a few minutes to allow the yeast to activate.

Meanwhile, add all the dry ingredients to an electric stand mixer (with dough hook attachment), and mix well. Then, add the yeast mixture, along with the olive oil, and mix at a medium speed. Knead the dough for 8 minutes. If your dough looks slightly too wet, add a little flour; if too dry, a touch more water.

Lightly grease a bowl with oil. Place the dough into the bowl and cover with a damp cloth. Leave it somewhere warm for 45 minutes, or until the dough has doubled in size.

For the tamarind sauce, add all the ingredients to a blender with 240ml (1 cup) water and blitz until smooth. Transfer to a small pan over a low heat to bubble away and thicken up for about 15 minutes. Once thick, the sauce is ready.

To make the cucumber salsa, simply mix all the ingredients together in a bowl.

Back to the baras. Lightly flour your work surface and remove the risen dough from the bowl. Roll the dough into a big sausage shape and cut it into 16 equal pieces. Roll each piece into a 1-cm (½-in) thick circle shape (around 13cm/5in in diameter). Lightly flour each one, then place them onto greaseproof paper.

Half-fill a large saucepan with the vegetable oil then place over a medium heat. When the oil is hot (test by dipping a wooden spoon into the oil – if the spoon bubbles, the oil is hot enough), carefully place one piece of dough into the oil and fry for 2 minutes on each side. Use a spider to carefully turn the bara over. Once golden and bubbly, remove the bara and place it onto a plate lined with kitchen paper, to soak up excess oil. Repeat for the rest of the dough, frying one bara at a time.

To serve, place two baras on a piece of greaseproof paper and top with a generous amount of the curry, tamarind sauce and cucumber salsa.

Pictured on page 87.

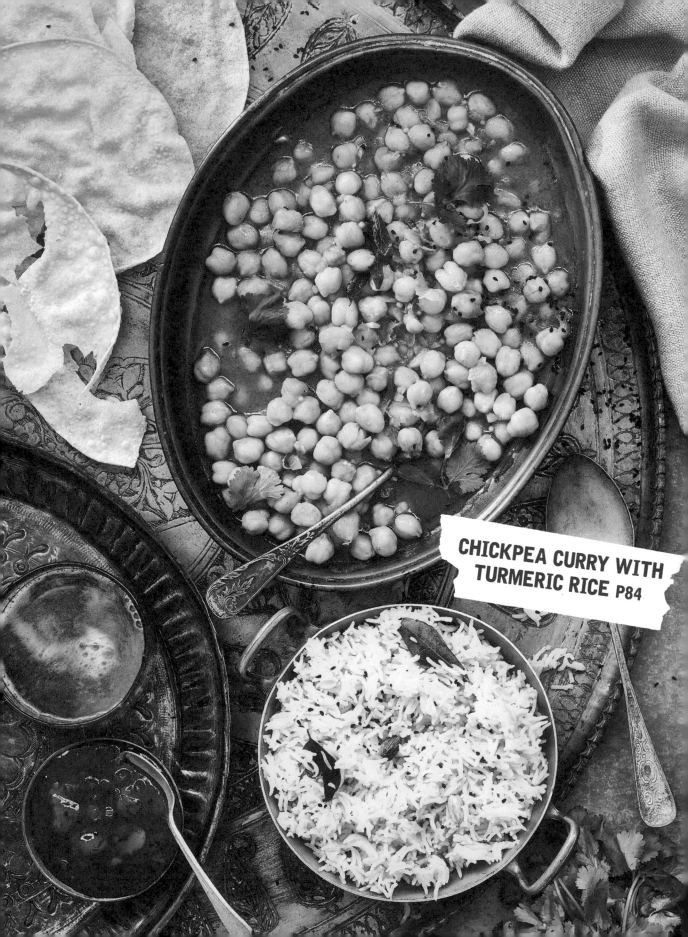

CHICKPEA CURRY WITH TURMERIC RICE P84

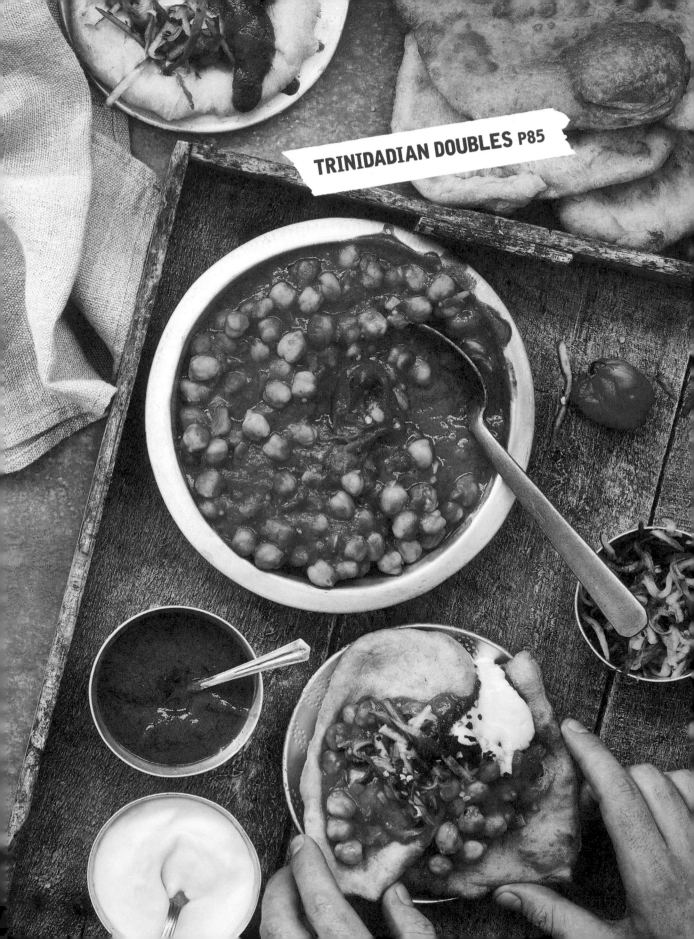

TRINIDADIAN DOUBLES P85

THAI GREEN CURRY

SERVES **4**	COOKS IN **40 MINS**	DIFFICULTY **5/10**

vegetable oil, for frying

1 x 280-g (10-oz) block firm tofu

½ butternut squash, peeled, cubed and steamed or boiled until tender

handful broccolini, each piece cut into 3 pieces

handful of mangetout (snow peas)

1 x 400-ml (14-fl oz) can coconut milk

for the curry paste

1 tsp cumin seeds

2 tsp coriander seeds

1 tsp sea salt

4 garlic cloves

1 lemongrass stem, woody part removed, finely chopped

thumb-sized piece of fresh ginger, peeled

juice of ½ lime

5 green bird's eye chillies

1 tsp soy sauce (or tamari for GF)

2 Kaffir lime leaves (fresh or dried)

handful of fresh coriander (cilantro)

to serve

freish Thai basil

rice or noodles

handful of coriander (cilantro)

lime wedges

1 red chilli, finely chopped

roasted peanuts (optional)

First up, make the curry paste. Start by toasting the cumin and coriander seeds. Place them in a dry frying pan (skillet) to toast over a medium heat, this won't take long – roughly 2 minutes. You will start smelling them; that's when you know they are ready.

Place the toasted seeds and all the remaining paste ingredients into a blender. Blitz until it forms a smooth paste. You may need to add a little vegetable oil or water to help the mixture blend.

To make the curry, cut the tofu into bite-sized cubes. You need to get the tofu and squash nicely coloured. Place a large saucepan or wok over a high heat and add a touch of oil. Add the tofu and squash and stir-fry for 3–4 minutes, stirring often, until they are nicely golden.

Add a generous tablespoon of the curry paste to the wok, toss the pan to get all the tofu nicely coated. Then throw in the rest of the vegetables.

Cook everything for a couple of minutes before deglazing the wok with the coconut milk and 240ml (1 cup) water (I usually use the coconut can to measure this). Turn the heat down to low and let the curry bubble away for around 10–12 minutes.

Serve your curry with rice or noodles and garnish each plate with some fresh Thai basil, coriander (cilantro), a wedge of lime, chopped red chilli and a little sprinkle of roasted peanuts for a nice crunch.

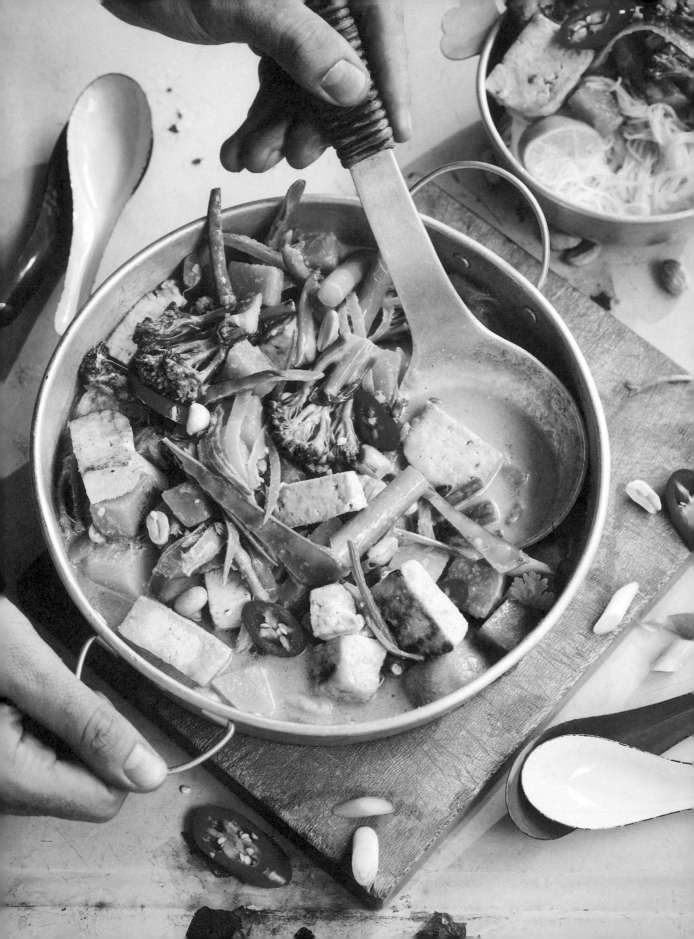

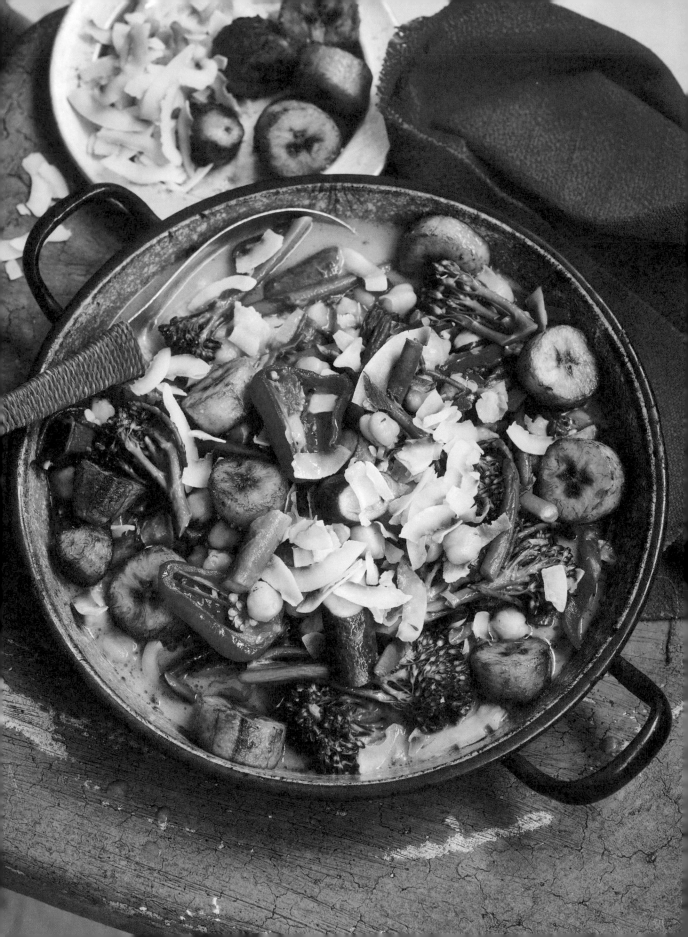

JAMAICAN VEGETABLE CURRY

Make sure you've got Scotch bonnet chillies to give this dish a real
authentic taste. This is my go-to curry, and best of all, it's ready in no time.

SERVES **4**	COOKS IN **15 MINS**	DIFFICULTY **3/10**

3 tbsp coconut oil

5 spring onions (scallions), finely chopped

5 garlic cloves, minced

1 Scotch bonnet, halved

1 tbsp dried thyme

1 bay leaf

2 tbsp Jamaican curry powder

½ tsp ground ginger

3 tbsp tomato purée

1 red (bell) pepper, sliced

5 baby courgettes (zucchini), chopped

handful of fine green beans, chopped

handful of broccolini, chopped

handful of asparagus tips

1 x 400-ml (14-fl oz) can coconut milk

1 x 400-g (14-oz) can chickpeas (garbanzos), drained and rinsed

handful of samphire (optional)

sea salt and ground black pepper

serve with

Fried Plantain (page 169)

toasted coconut flakes

Heat a large non-stick pan or a wok over a medium heat. Add the coconut oil, followed by the spring onions (scallions), garlic, chilli and a pinch of salt and pepper. Sauté for 1 minute before adding the dried herbs, spices and the tomato purée. Cook the mixture, stirring often, for 4–5 minutes.

Add the (bell) pepper, courgette (zucchini), fine beans, broccolini and asparagus. Allow to cook for a few minutes, mixing well, so everything gets coated in the lovely flavours.

Deglaze the pan by adding the coconut milk, chickpeas (garbanzos) and 240ml (1 cup) water. Turn the heat up and allow the curry to bubble away for a few minutes to thicken up, before adding the samphire, if using.

Once thickened, go ahead and serve. Scatter some Fried Plantain over the top, as well as a sprinkle of toasted coconut flakes.

HOT & FRUITY INDIAN CHICK'N CURRY PIE

Fruit in curries work so well, especially in spicy curries. The apple in this recipe gives it such a zing, in among all the wonderful spices. I like to use a pie chimney – it allows the air to escape and looks so cool! With its crispy, flaky pastry, this is a real show stopper!

SERVES **4–6**	COOKS IN **80 MINS**	DIFFICULTY **5/10**

3 tbsp vegetable oil

2 cardamon pods

4 fresh or dried curry leaves

1 cinnamon stick

1 green chilli, halved lengthwise

1 onion, finely chopped

5 garlic cloves, minced

1 tbsp minced fresh root ginger

1 tsp mustard seeds

½ tsp ground turmeric

2 tsp chilli powder

1 tsp ground cumin

1 tsp ground coriander

pinch nutmeg

2 tsp sea salt

2 tbsp tomato purée

200g (2 cups) vegan 'chicken', or vegan protein of your choice

2 apples, peeled and cubed

1 x 400-g (14-oz) can chopped tomatoes

handful of chopped coriander (cilantro)

500g (18oz) block of ready-to-roll puff pastry

plain (all-purpose) flour or gluten-free flour, for dusting

for the glaze

2 tbsp maple syrup

2 tbsp olive oil

2 tbsp non-dairy milk

Sprinkle black onion seeds over the pie before serving. They have a delicious aromatic flavour.

Method on page 94...

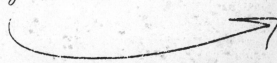

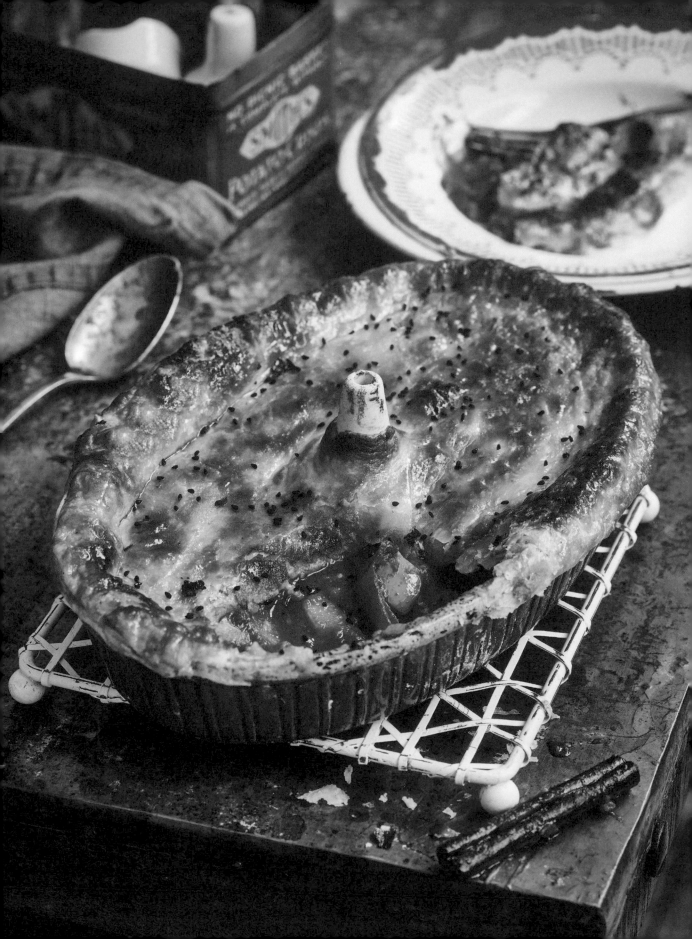

Hot & Fruity Indian Chick'n Curry Pie method...

Place a large non-stick saucepan over a low heat and add the oil. When hot, add the cardamon pods, curry leaves, cinnamon stick and the green chilli. Allow them to infuse the oil and release their flavours for a couple of minutes before adding the onion, garlic and ginger, then let everything cook for 10 minutes. It's important to let the onions turn nice and golden – this will release all their sugars, resulting in a lovely base flavour to your curry.

Once the onions are golden, add all the remaining spices and the sea salt. Cook for a couple of minutes, stirring often.

Add the tomato purée, vegan 'chicken' and the apple. Stir well, so the chicken and apple are coated in all the beautiful flavours.

Add the chopped tomatoes and about 240ml (1 cup) water – I just swill the tomato can out with water and add that. Mix well, then place a lid on the saucepan and let the curry simmer away for 20 minutes, stirring every now and then.

After 20 minutes the curry should have thickened up, smell beautiful and the apples softened. Turn off the heat to let the curry cool slightly.

Before assembling your pie, preheat your oven to 180°C (350°F).

On a lightly floured work surface, roll out your pastry to about 2.5cm (1in) bigger than your baking dish and around 3mm (⅛in) thick.

Mix the glaze ingredients together in a small bowl.

Spoon the curry into your baking dish and top with the pastry. Crimp the edges with your fingers and brush the glaze over. I like to make a little incision in the middle of the pastry using a knife and insert a pie chimney so the air has somewhere to escape when the pie is cooking – but it's not essential.

Pop the pie into the oven on the middle shelf to bake for 30 minutes. Once the pastry has puffed up and is lovely and golden, serve up.

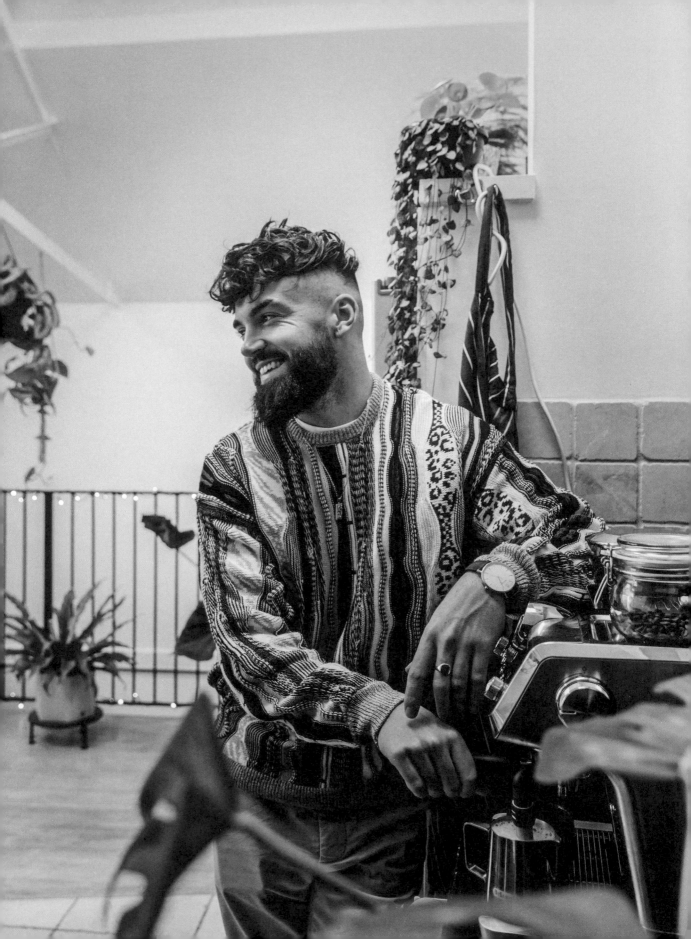

PUNCHY PEANUT CURRY

I often use this hearty curry for my meal preps. Baking the tofu before adding it to the curry helps to make it super meaty. Swap out the peanut butter for tahini to make it nut-free, and to make it oil-free, sauté the vegetables in water.

SERVES **4–6**	COOKS IN **50 MINS**	DIFFICULTY **3/10**

1 tbsp olive oil (optional)

2 red onions, cut into chunks

3 garlic cloves, minced

thumb-sized piece of fresh ginger, peeled and minced

1 red chilli, deseeded and finely chopped

1 tbsp curry powder

1 tbsp dried thyme

2 tsp sea salt

1 small butternut squash, peeled and deseeded, then cubed

1 red (bell) pepper, diced

2 tbsp tomato purée

1 x 280g (10oz) block firm tofu, cubed

2 tbsp crunchy peanut butter

1 x 400ml (14fl oz) can coconut milk

handful of coriander (cilantro), roughly chopped

to serve

rice

spring onions (scallions), chopped

lime wedges

Preheat your oven to 180°C (350°F) and line a baking sheet with baking paper.

Place a large non stick saucepan over a medium heat. Add the oil (if using), followed by the onion, garlic, ginger and chilli. Sauté the mixture for 4 minutes, making sure you get the onions lovely and golden. Add the curry powder, thyme and salt, then cook for a couple of minutes more.

Turn the heat down to low, then add the squash, pepper, tomato purée and 240ml (1 cup) water. Pop a lid on the pan and cook for at least 12 minutes or until the squash is tender. Give it a stir every couple of minutes.

Meanwhile, pat the tofu cubes dry using kitchen paper. Place the cubes onto the lined baking sheet, then bake in the oven for 15 minutes.

Once the squash is tender, stir in the peanut butter and coconut milk.

Your tofu should be golden and 'meaty' now, so remove it from the oven and stir it through the curry, along with the chopped coriander (cilantro).

Let the curry bubble away for a further 10 minutes. Taste for seasoning and add additional water if the curry is too thick for your liking.

Serve the curry with rice, garnished with chopped spring onions (scallions) and lime wedges.

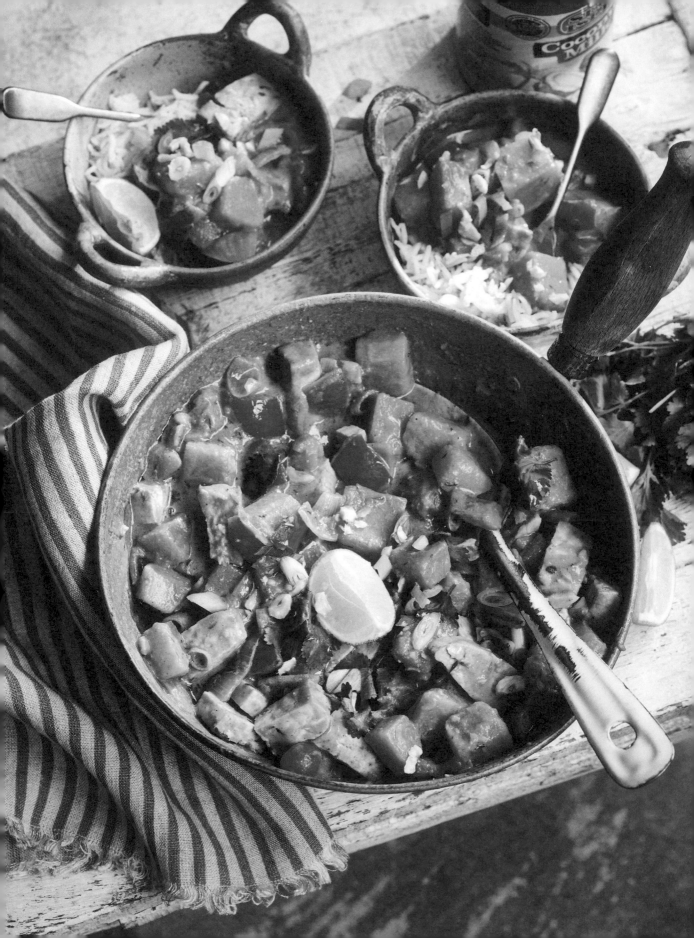

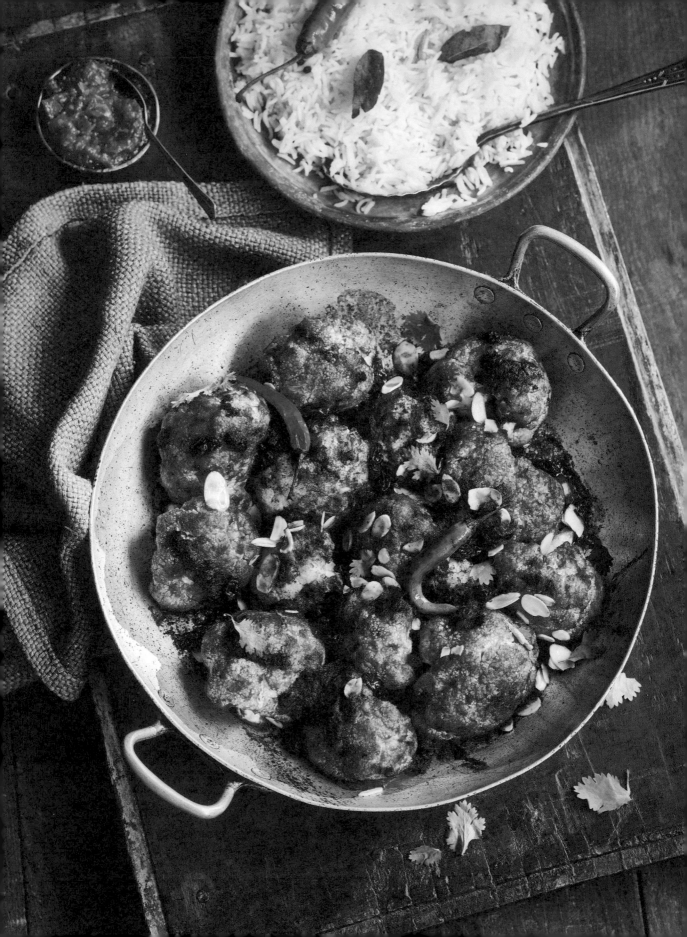

ROASTED CURRIED CAULIFLOWER

SERVES **4**	COOKS IN **45 MINS**	DIFFICULTY **5/10**

1 white onion, roughly chopped

4 garlic cloves

2 green chillies

3 tbsp tomato purée

1 tsp ground turmeric

1 tsp ground cumin

1 tsp ground coriander

1 tsp ground mace

1 tsp ground fenugreek

1 tsp sea salt

1 tbsp olive oil

2 cauliflowers, outer leaves removed, cut into large florets

3 tbsp flaked (slivered) almonds

3 tbsp sultanas (golden raisins) or raisins

to serve

fresh coriander (cilantro)

rice

lime pickle

Preheat your oven to 190°C (375°F).

First up, you will need to make a beautiful aromatic curry paste. Add the onion, garlic, chilli, tomato purée, all the spices and salt to a blender. Give it a pulse, then add enough water to help it blend into a smooth-ish paste.

Heat a large oven-proof frying pan (skillet) over a medium heat and add the oil. When hot, add the curry paste, and cook for 4–5 minutes before adding the cauliflower florets.

Allow the cauliflower to colour for a couple of minutes, then sprinkle over the flaked (slivered) almonds and sultanas (golden raisins) or raisins.

Turn the heat off, then carefully cover the pan with foil. Place the pan into the oven on the bottom shelf for 30 minutes.

After 25 minutes of cooking, remove the foil so that the cauliflower colours nicely on top, adding a lovely flavour.

After 30 minutes, check your cauliflower is tender by poking a small knife or skewer into one of the pieces. If they are a little hard, simply put them back into the oven for a little longer.

Serve up the cauliflower with a sprinkle of chopped coriander (cilantro), rice and some lime pickle.

I like to use a cast-iron pan for this recipe. If you don't have an oven-proof pan, you can still make this recipe — just make sure you have a baking dish at the ready to transfer the mixture into before it goes into the oven.

SIMPLE CHINESE CURRY

SERVES 4–6	COOKS IN **45 MINS**	DIFFICULTY **3/10**

vegetable oil, for frying

2 white onions, cut into chunks

4 garlic cloves, minced

1 red chilli, finely sliced

thumb-sized piece of fresh ginger, peeled and finely chopped

3 tsp curry powder

3 tsp Chinese five spice

2 tsp sea salt

1 tsp cracked black pepper

1 green (bell) pepper, deseeded and diced

1 carrot, thinly sliced

250g (9oz) mixed Asian mushrooms

2 x 400-g (14-oz) cans jackfruit, drained and water squeezed out

1 litre (1¾ pints) vegetable stock

1 x 160-ml (5½-fl oz) can coconut cream

2 tsp lemongrass paste

1 tbsp miso paste

to serve

4 spring onions (scallions), finely chopped

1 red chilli, finely chopped

wholewheat noodles, cooked according to packet instructions

Place a large saucepan over a medium heat and add a touch of oil. When the pan is hot add the onion, garlic, chilli, ginger, curry powder, Chinese five spice, salt and pepper.

Fry the mixture for 2–3 minutes, stirring often, before adding the (bell) pepper, carrot, mushrooms and jackfruit. Keep frying for a further 5 minutes, getting the mushrooms nice and golden.

Deglaze the pan with the stock, coconut cream, lemongrass and miso paste.

Pop a lid on, turn the heat down and let the curry bubble away for 30 minutes. Stir every now and then.

When the curry has thickened nicely it is ready to serve.

Sprinkle over the chopped spring onions (scallions) and chilli before serving with noodles.

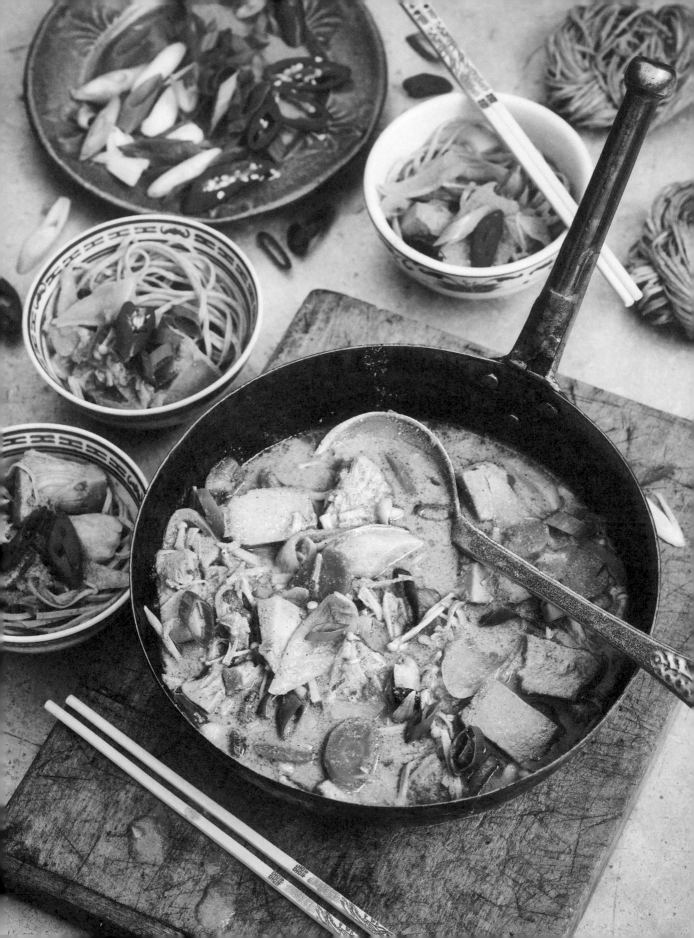

06

Big Plates

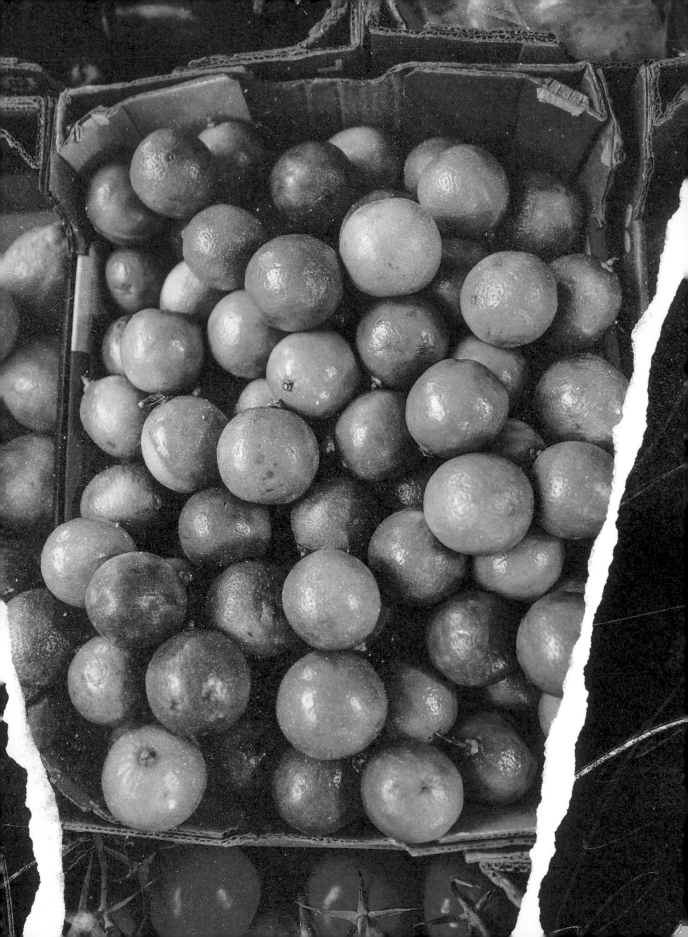

NASI GORENG

I fell in love with the nasi goreng I tried on a trip to Indonesia, and I love my version just as much. It's so simple and quick to make. 'Nasi goreng' simply means 'fried rice'. Any left over sambal can be stored in a sealed container in the fridge for a couple of weeks, making it even quicker to make next time.

SERVES **4**	COOKS IN **20 MINS**	DIFFICULTY **5/10**

360g (2 cups) long-grain rice

1 red onion, finely sliced

125g (1 cup) frozen peas, defrosted

1 red (bell) pepper, finely sliced

5 baby courgettes (zucchini), sliced at an angle

handful of fine beans, chopped

175–190g (1 cup) vegan protein, such as tofu cubes or vegan 'chicken'

3 tbsp kecap manis or soy sauce

handful of toasted cashew nuts

for the crispy shallots

2 shallots, finely sliced

500ml (2 cups) vegetable oil

pinch sea salt

for the sambal

3 red chillies

3 garlic cloves

1 tbsp tomato purée

1 tbsp lemongrass paste

2 tbsp groundnut oil

1 tsp sea salt

juice and zest of 1 lime

First up, get your rice cooking, according to the packet instructions.

To make the crispy shallots, simply heat a small pan half-filled with vegetable oil to around 180°C (350°F). Or, dip a wooden spoon into the oil; if bubbles form around the wood, your oil is hot enough. Carefully lower in the shallots and fry for 2 minutes, or until golden. Remove the shallots from the oil and place onto a plate lined with kitchen paper, to drain off any excess oil.

Add all the sambal ingredients to a blender and blitz to a smooth paste.

Preheat a wok over a high heat, then add the sambal. Cook for a minute or so, stirring often.

Add all the vegetables and vegan protein to the wok and stir-fry for 5–6 minutes.

When your rice is cooked, drain and add the rice to the wok. Stir-fry for 3–4 minutes. Be sure to mix well and stir often, so the rice doesn't stick and burn.

Stir in the kecap manis or soy sauce and the cashew nuts. When the rice is beautifully coated in all the flavours, turn off the heat and serve up with a sprinkle of the crispy shallots.

Pictured on pages 106–7.

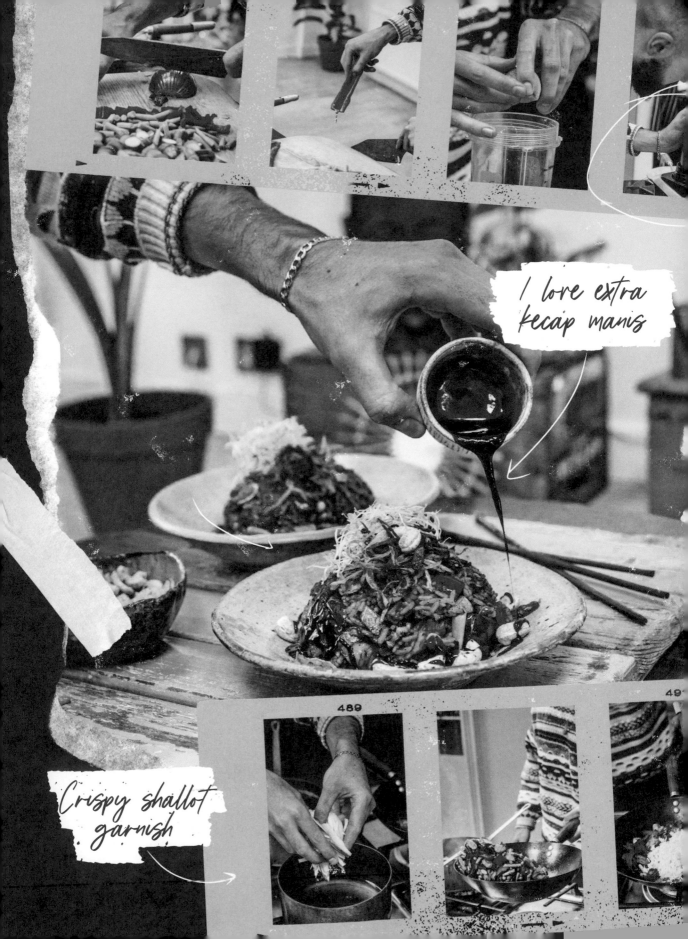

I love extra kecap manis

Crispy shallot garnish

489

49

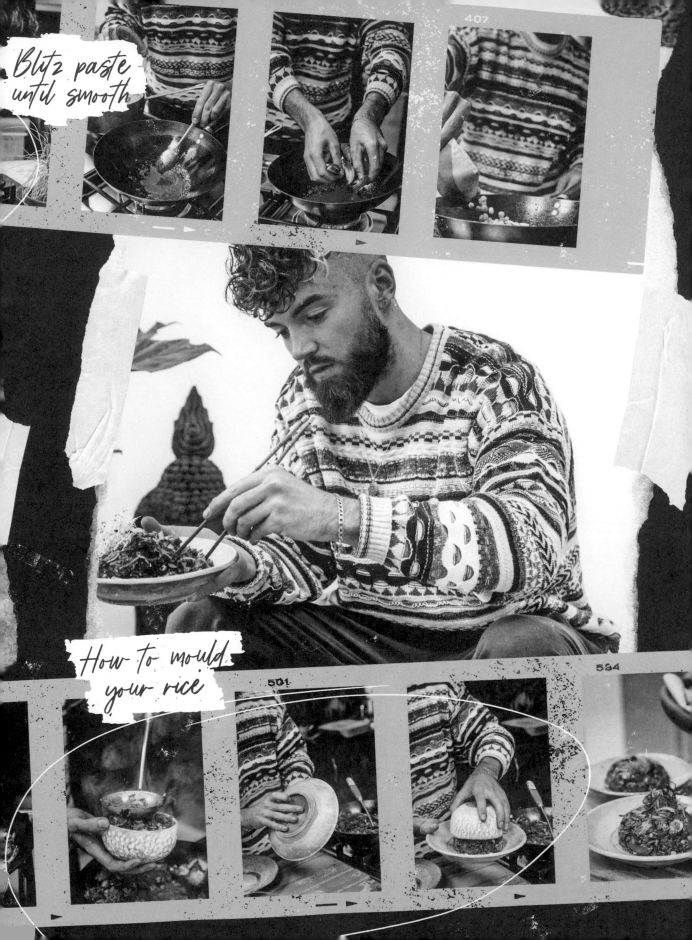

Blitz paste until smooth

407

How to mould your rice

501

594

CRISPY FRIED LEMON TOFU

| SERVES **4** | COOKS IN **30 MINS** | DIFFICULTY **5/10** |

270g (2 cups) self-raising flour or gluten-free flour

1 tsp baking powder

1 tsp sea salt, plus extra for sprinkling

480ml (2 cups) lemon kombucha or sparkling water

1 litre (1¾ pints) vegetable oil, for frying

2 x 280-g (10-oz) packs firm tofu, patted dry and cubed

1 onion, quartered

½ head of broccoli, cut into florets

1 red (bell) pepper, finely sliced

5 spring onions (scallions), cut into 2-cm (¾-in) pieces

2 pak choi (bok choy), quartered

1 cup frozen peas

for the lemon sauce

zest and juice of 2 lemons

2 tbsp rice wine vinegar

3 tbsp caster (superfine) sugar

1 tbsp soy sauce or tamari

2 tsp Sriracha sauce

2 tbsp cornflour (cornstarch)

to serve

boiled rice

toasted cashew nuts

Mushroom 'Prawn' Toasts (page 61)

First, make the lemon sauce. Add all the ingredients, apart from the cornflour (cornstarch), to a small saucepan along with 360ml (3 cups) water and mix. Place the saucepan over a low heat and allow to simmer for 10 minutes, stirring every now and then.

Meanwhile, place the cornflour in a small bowl and mix with enough water to make a smooth runny consistency.

Whisk the cornflour mixture into the sauce, and continue to whisk until the sauce has thickened up. Add a touch more water if it thickens too much or little more cornflour if it's too thin. Set the sauce aside until you're ready to serve. (The sauce can be stored in a sealed container in the fridge for up to 3 weeks.)

To make the crispy tofu, add the flour, baking powder and salt to a bowl and mix thoroughly. Whisk in enough kombucha or sparkling water until you have a pancake-batter consistency.

Half-fill a large saucepan with the oil and heat over a medium heat to 180°C (350°F). Or dip a wooden spoon in the oil and if bubbles form around it, the oil is hot enough.

Carefully dip the tofu cubes into the batter before gently lowering them into the hot oil. Fry the tofu cubes for 3 minutes or until they are golden and crisp. Flip them over half-way through cooking using a spider or slotted spoon.

Remove the crispy tofu from the oil and place onto a plate lined with kitchen paper. Sprinkle with salt and set aside until you're ready to serve.

Heat a large wok over a high heat and add a touch of oil. When hot, add the onion, broccoli, (bell) pepper, spring onions (scallions), pak choi (bok choy) and peas and stir-fry for 5 minutes, adding a touch of the lemon sauce towards the end of frying.

Serve the vegetables with rice, the crispy tofu balls, a handful of toasted cashew nuts and lots of sauce, with Mushroom 'Prawn' Toasts on the side.

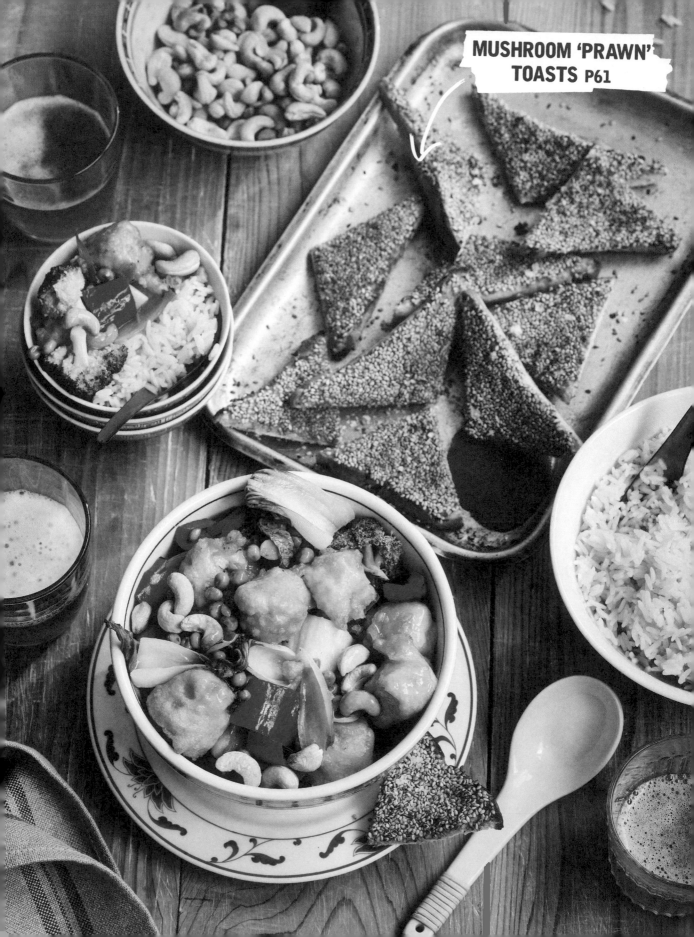

MUSHROOM 'PRAWN' TOASTS P61

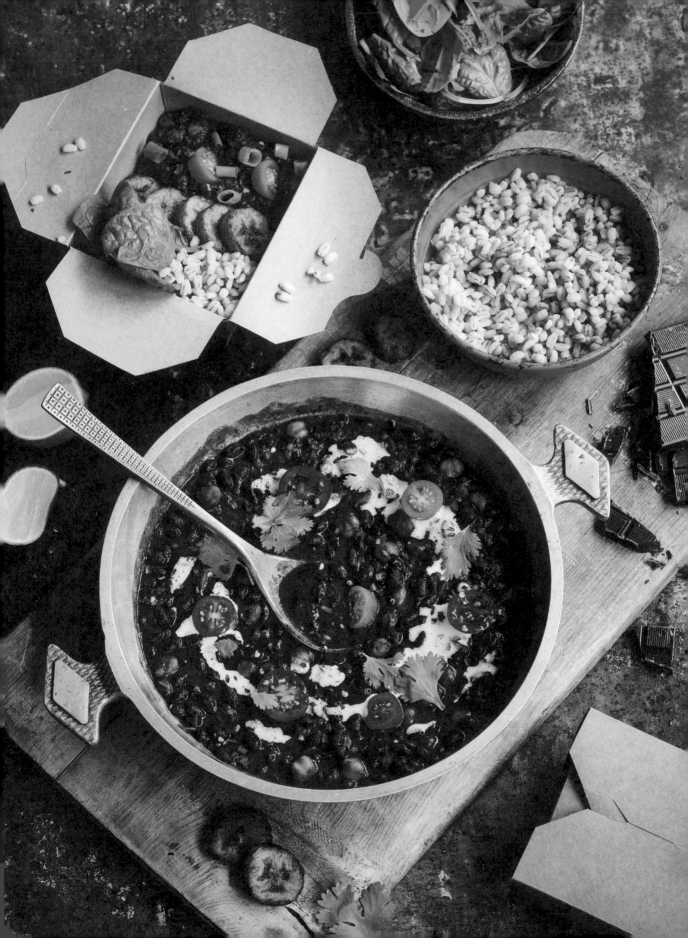

BLACK BEAN STEW WITH PEARL BARLEY

SERVES **4**	COOKS IN **35 MINS**	DIFFICULTY **3/10**

2 tbsp vegetable oil

1 red onion, finely chopped

3 garlic cloves, minced

1 fresh chilli, finely chopped

2 tsp sea salt

1 tsp ground coriander

2 tsp ground cumin

½ tsp ground cinnamon

2 tsp dried oregano

2 tsp dried thyme

2 tbsp chipotle paste

2 x 400-g (14-oz) cans black beans, drained and rinsed

1 x 400-g (14-oz) can chickpeas (garbanzos), drained and rinsed

2 tbsp tomato purée

2 tbsp soy sauce (or tamari for GF)

juice of 1 lime

1 tbsp dairy-free dark chocolate, chopped

handful of chopped coriander (cilantro), plus extra for serving

handful of cherry tomatoes, halved, to serve

vegan yogurt, to serve

for the pearl barley

300g (1½ cups) pearl barley

zest and juice of 1 lime

pinch each sea salt and pepper

Preheat a saucepan over a medium heat and add the oil, followed by the onion, garlic, chilli and salt. Sauté until softened.

Add the dried spices and herbs, then cook for 3–4 minutes, stirring often. Next, add the chipotle paste and black beans, followed by 480ml (2 cups) water, the tomato puree, soy sauce and lime juice.

Place a lid on the pan and simmer for around 20 minutes or until the lovely liquid has thickened up.

Meanwhile, cook the pearl barley according to the packet instructions. Once cooked, simply mix through the lime zest, juice, and seasoning.

Just before serving, stir the chocolate and chopped coriander (cilantro) through the stew.

Serve up the stew garnished with a handful of cherry tomatoes, a few coriander (cilantro) leaves and a drizzle of vegan yogurt, alongside the barley.

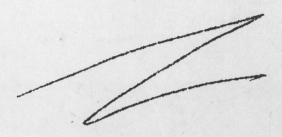

JERK JACKFRUIT WITH RICE & PEAS

SERVES **4-6**	COOKS IN **45 MINS**	DIFFICULTY **5/10**

3 x 400-g (14-oz) cans young jackfruit in brine, drained

1 tbsp coconut oil

3 spring onions (scallions), finely sliced

3 garlic cloves, minced

thumb-sized piece of fresh ginger, peeled and minced

½ Scotch bonnet chilli, finely chopped

1 yellow (bell) pepper, diced

1 tbsp allspice

2 tsp ground cinnamon

4 tbsp coconut sugar

200g (1 cup) canned black beans, drained and rinsed

3 tbsp soy sauce

5 tbsp tomato purée

240ml (1 cup) pineapple juice

juice of 1 lime

1 tbsp fresh thyme leaves, chopped

sea salt and black pepper

for the rice and peas

1 x 400-g (14-oz) can kidney beans, drained, liquid reserved

1 x 400-ml (14-fl oz) can coconut milk

3 tbsp fresh thyme

pinch sea salt and black pepper

340g (1½ cups) long-grain rice, washed

to serve

Tostones (page 168)

lime wedges

salad

Put the jackfruit into the middle of a clean kitchen (dish) towel. Pick up the corners of the towel, then squeeze out the liquid over a sink by twisting the towel. Getting rid of water will ensure the jackfruit has a meaty texture.

Place a large casserole dish or frying pan (skillet) over a medium heat. Add the coconut oil, followed by the spring onions (scallions), garlic, ginger, chilli and yellow (bell) pepper. Allow the mixture to soften for 3 minutes before adding the spices. Cook for 2 minutes, then add a pinch of seasoning. Add the jackfruit to the pan and stir well. Cook the mixture for a further 3–4 minutes.

Next, add the coconut sugar and the black beans. Keep stirring, then add the soy sauce, tomato purée and pineapple juice. Turn the heat down to low and add the lime juice and the chopped thyme. Pop the lid on and allow the jackfruit to cook for around 12–15 minutes, stirring every now and then.

For the rice and peas, add all the ingredients to a pan and cover. Place over a low heat and allow the rice to absorb the liquid until it's light and fluffy. This should take 10–12 minutes. If it gets too dry before it has cooked, add water.

Serve the cooked jackfruit with the rice and peas immediately with Tostones, lime wedges and a salad on the side.

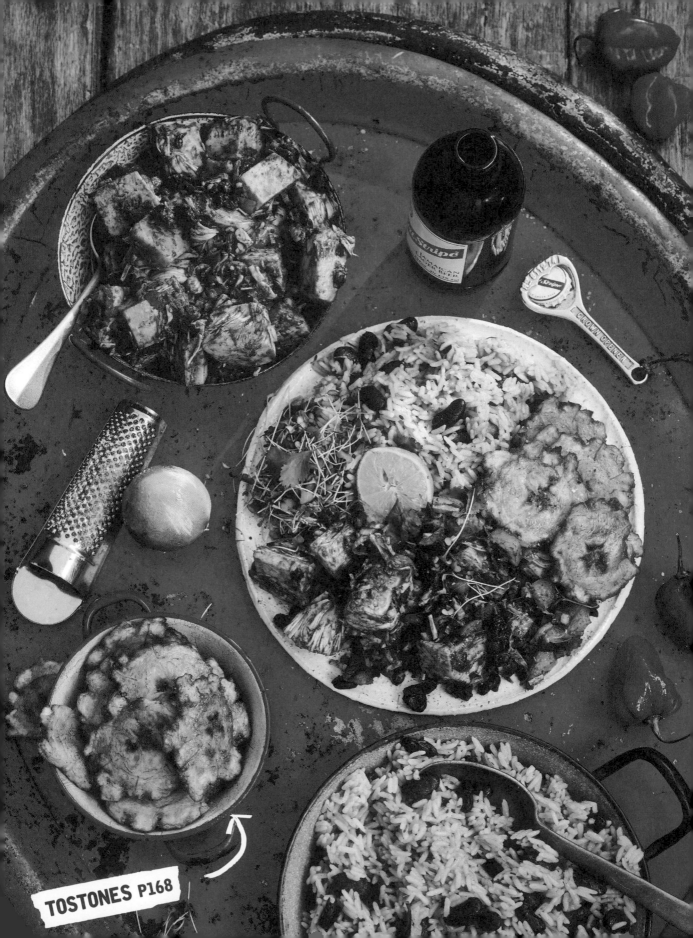

TOSTONES P168

THE RAMEN

| SERVES **4-6** | COOKS IN **90 MINS** | DIFFICULTY **5/10** |

for the broth

2 tbsp vegetable oil

1 onion, cut into 8 pieces

3 garlic cloves, roughly chopped

250g (9oz) shiitake mushrooms

4 ripe tomatoes

thumb-sized piece of fresh ginger, peeled and minced

2 green chillies

1.5 litres (2½ pints) vegetable stock

1 star anise

1 cinnamon stick

5 whole peppercorns

5 tbsp soy sauce or tamari

2 tbsp rice vinegar

for the coated tofu

3 tbsp miso paste

1 tbsp sesame oil

2 tbsp maple syrup

70g (½ cup) mixed sesame seeds

1 x 280-g (10-oz) block firm tofu, water pressed out

to serve

cooked noodles of your choice

a selection of fresh vegetables, such as: quartered baby pak choi (bok choy), sliced carrot, sugarsnap peas, spring onions (scallions), beansprouts and enoki mushrooms

First, make the broth. Place a large saucepan over a low heat and add the oil, followed by the onion, garlic, mushrooms, tomatoes, ginger and chilli.

Sauté the mixture, stirring often, for 12–15 minutes. You want to get everything beautifully golden so that all the natural sugars and umami flavours are released – this will give you an incredible broth.

Deglaze the pan with the vegetable stock, then add all the remaining broth ingredients and stir well.

Let the broth simmer away for at least 30 minutes, then taste it. The longer you leave it the more the flavours will intensify, so just keep tasting it. When you love it, it's ready to serve!

Prepare the tofu by cutting the block into 16 rectangles. Preheat your oven to 180°C (350°F) and line a baking sheet with baking paper.

In a small bowl, mix together the miso, sesame oil and maple syrup with 4 tablespoons of water. The mix needs to be quite runny, if it's too thick then it's going to be very difficult to coat the tofu, so add a little extra water if needed. Put the sesame seeds in another bowl.

Individually dip the tofu rectangles first into the miso mix and then into the sesame seeds. Coat them as best as you can, then place the coated pieces onto your lined baking sheet. Once you've coated all the tofu, pop the tray into the oven for 25 minutes.

Once the tofu is baked and nicely golden brown, remove from the oven, ready to serve. I like to slice the pieces on an angle.

Build your ramen bowls. First put some noodles into each bowl, followed by a ladleful of the broth, then the vegetables and the sliced coated tofu.

Alternatively, if you don't want to cook all of the sesame tofu, you can place them in a container and freeze for another time.

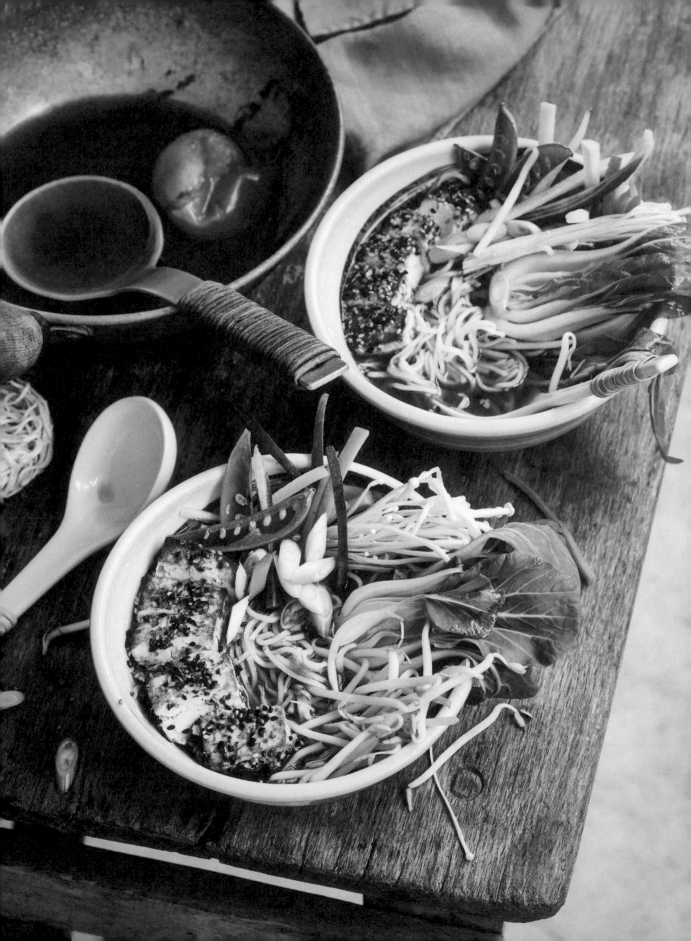

STICKY UMAMI EGGPLANTS

I guarantee this will convert anyone into an aubergine (eggplant) lover!
If you can't find baby aubergines, cut normal ones into chunks.

SERVES **4**	COOKS IN **15 MINS**	DIFFICULTY **3/10**

15 MIN · CAN BE GF · MEAL PREP

1 tbsp olive oil

8 baby aubergines (eggplants) cut in half lengthways (or 2 regular ones, cut into wedges)

2 shallots, finely sliced

3 garlic cloves, finely sliced

pinch each sea salt and pepper

1 tsp dried rosemary

3 tbsp balsamic vinegar

3 tbsp soy sauce or coconut aminos (for soy-free)

3 tbsp maple syrup

1 tbsp English mustard

for the lentils

1 x 400-g (14-oz) can green lentils, drained

zest and juice of 1 lemon

handful of chopped fresh herbs (I used mint, basil and parsley)

pinch each sea salt and pepper

handful of black olives

to serve

samphire, steamed (optional)

Heat the oil in a non-stick frying pan (skillet) over a medium heat. Place the aubergines (eggplants) into the pan, cut-side down, then add the shallots, garlic and seasoning.

Cook for 2–3 minutes, until the aubergines are nice and golden, then flip over. Add the rosemary, vinegar, soy sauce, maple syrup, mustard and 240ml (1 cup) water.

Turn the heat down and allow the liquid to reduce down to a glaze-like consistency for about 5 minutes.

Meanwhile, mix all the lentil ingredients together in a saucepan, and place over a low heat to warm up gently.

Once the aubergines are glazed, serve with the lentils and steamed samphire, if using.

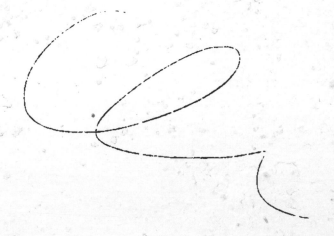

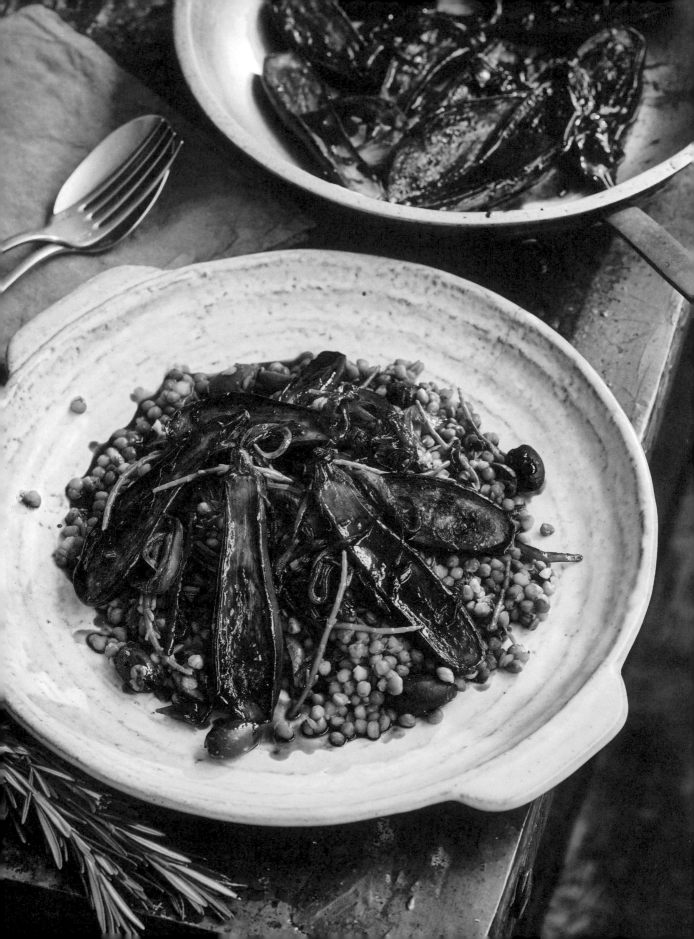

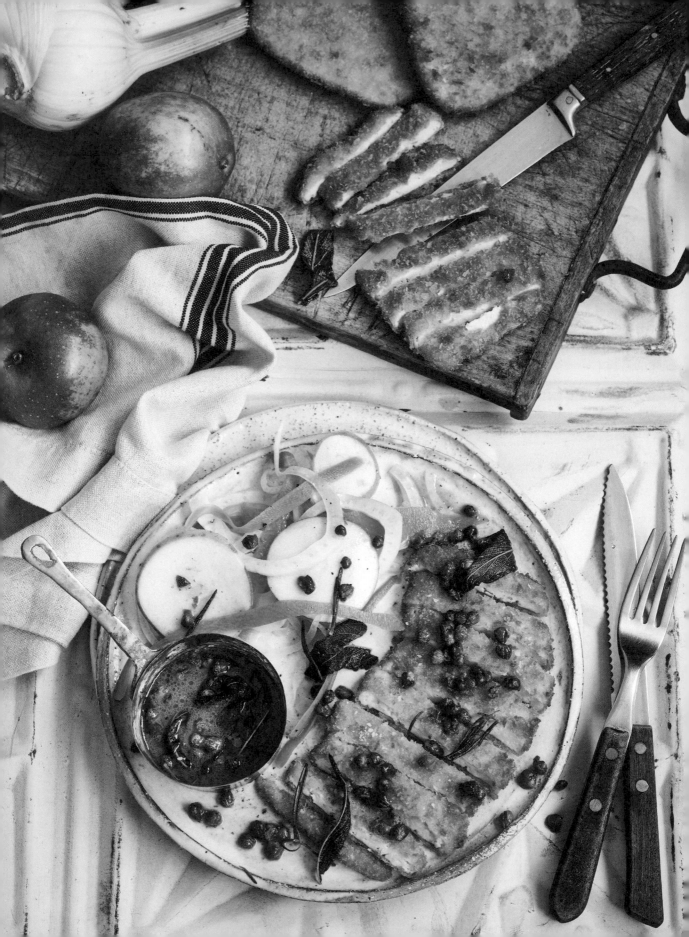

SCHNITZELS WITH HERB & CAPER SAUCE

| SERVES **4–6** | COOKS IN **45 MINS** | DIFFICULTY **5/10** |

1 x 480-g (17-oz) block firm tofu, sliced into 1-cm (½-in) slices

130g (1 cup) plain (all-purpose) flour or gluten-free flour

4 tbsp chicken seasoning

125g (1 cup) chickpea (gram) flour

100g (2 cups) panko breadcrumbs

120ml (½ cup) vegetable oil, for shallow frying

sea salt

for the slaw

1 apple, finely sliced on a mandoline or grated

1 carrot, finely sliced on a mandoline or grated

1 small fennel bulb, finely sliced on a mandoline or grated

juice of 1 lemon

pinch each sea salt and pepper

for the herb & caper sauce

5 tbsp vegan margarine

3 tbsp olive oil

1 banana shallot, finely chopped

juice of 1 lemon

4 tbsp capers

2 rosemary sprigs, leaves removed

small handful of sage leaves

First up, coat the tofu slices. Mix together the plain (all-purpose) flour and chicken seasoning in a bowl. In another bowl, whisk together the chickpea (gram) flour with enough water to make a beaten-egg-like consistency. Place the panko breadcrumbs in a third bowl. Line a baking sheet with greaseproof paper.

Individually dip each slice of tofu first into the dry flour mix, then the wet gram flour mix and finally the panko breadcrumbs. Once coated, place the tofu slices onto the lined baking sheet.

Preheat your oven to 180°C (350°F).

Place a large non-stick frying pan (skillet) over a medium heat and add the oil. When hot, shallow fry a few schnitzels at a time for around 2–3 minutes on each side. Once the schnitzels are nice and golden, place them back onto your lined baking sheet. When you've fried all of the schnitzels, place them into the oven to finish off cooking for 10 minutes.

Meanwhile, make the slaw. Simply mix all the sliced ingredients in a mixing bowl and squeeze over the lemon juice. Season with salt and pepper, then set aside until you're ready to serve.

Just before serving, make the herb and caper sauce. Place a small non-stick frying pan (skillet) over a medium heat. Add the margarine and oil and, when the margarine has melted, add the shallot and allow it sweat it down for a minute or so. Add the rest of the ingredients and allow the sauce to cook away for a couple of minutes. Add a couple of drops of water to loosen the sauce slightly.

Serve the schnitzels sprinkled with a little sea salt, with plenty of slaw, and the sauce drizzled over the top.

Chicken seasoning is a spice blend that's available from supermarkets. It doesn't actually contain chicken!

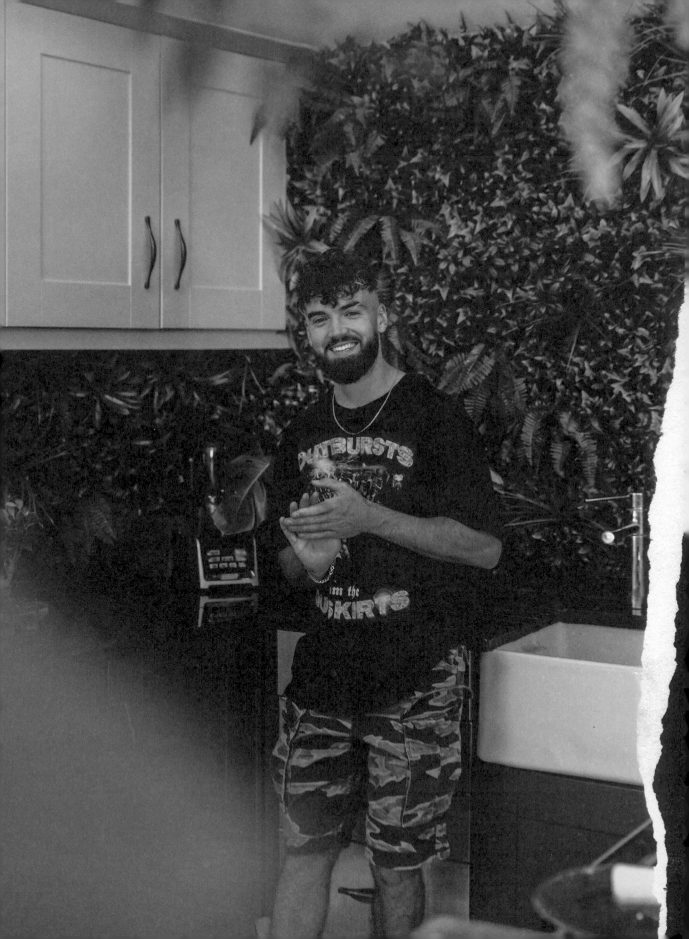

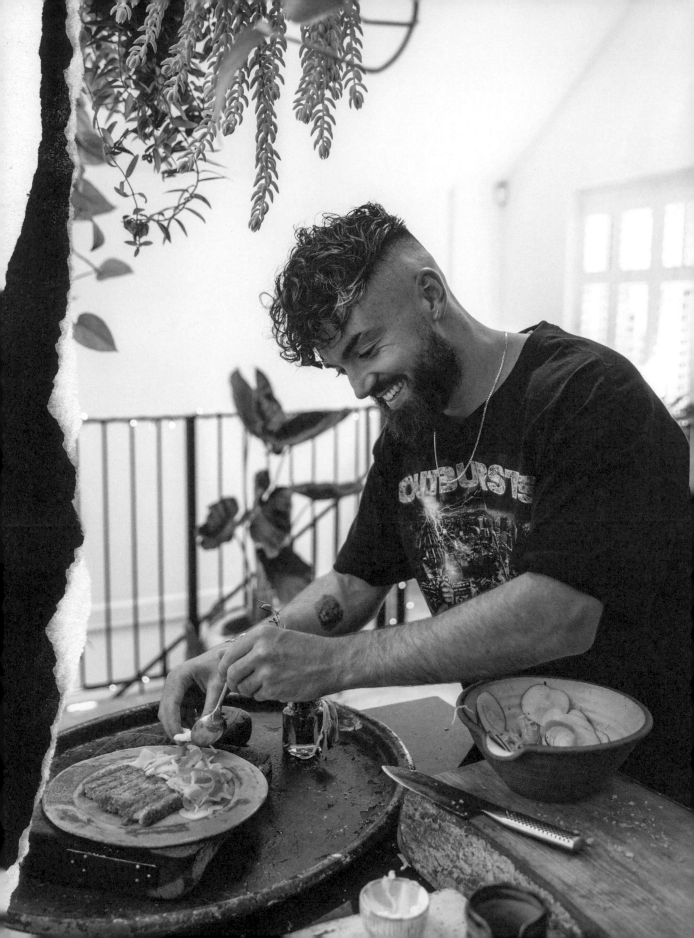

JACKFRUIT CAKES WITH ANCHO SAUCE

SERVES **4–6**	COOKS IN **90 MINS**	DIFFICULTY **7/10**

CAN
BE
GF

2 x 400-g (14-oz) cans young jackfruit, drained

5 spring onions (scallions), finely chopped

4 garlic cloves, minced

3 tbsp chipotle paste

1 tsp sea salt

1 tsp cracked black pepper

handful of chopped coriander (cilantro)

juice of 1 lime

2 tbsp plain (all-purpose) flour, or gluten-free flour for dusting

100g (2 cups) panko breadcrumbs

125g (1 cup) chickpea (gram) flour

2 tsp paprika

2 tsp dried thyme

vegetable oil, for frying

for the ancho sauce

3 dried ancho chillies

1 onion, diced

3 garlic cloves, peeled

240ml (1 cup) vegetable stock

1 tbsp dried thyme

2 tsp ground cinnamon

1 tsp ground cumin

1 tbsp coconut sugar or caster (superfine) sugar

1 tsp sea salt

1 x 400-g (14-oz) can black beans, drained and rinsed

2 tbsp chopped dark dairy-free chocolate

to serve

Grilled Baby Gem Lettuce in Orange Sauce (page 174)

Line a baking sheet with greaseproof paper. Preheat your oven to 180°C (350°F).

Put the jackfruit into the middle of a clean kitchen (dish) towel. Pick up the corners of the towel then squeeze the liquid from the jackfruit over your sink by twisting the towel. Getting rid of as much water as possible is important to ensure your jackfruit has a meaty texture.

Transfer the jackfruit to a mixing bowl, then add the spring onions (scallions), garlic, chipotle paste, sea salt, pepper, coriander (cilantro) and lime, then mix really well using your hands.

Method continued on page 129...

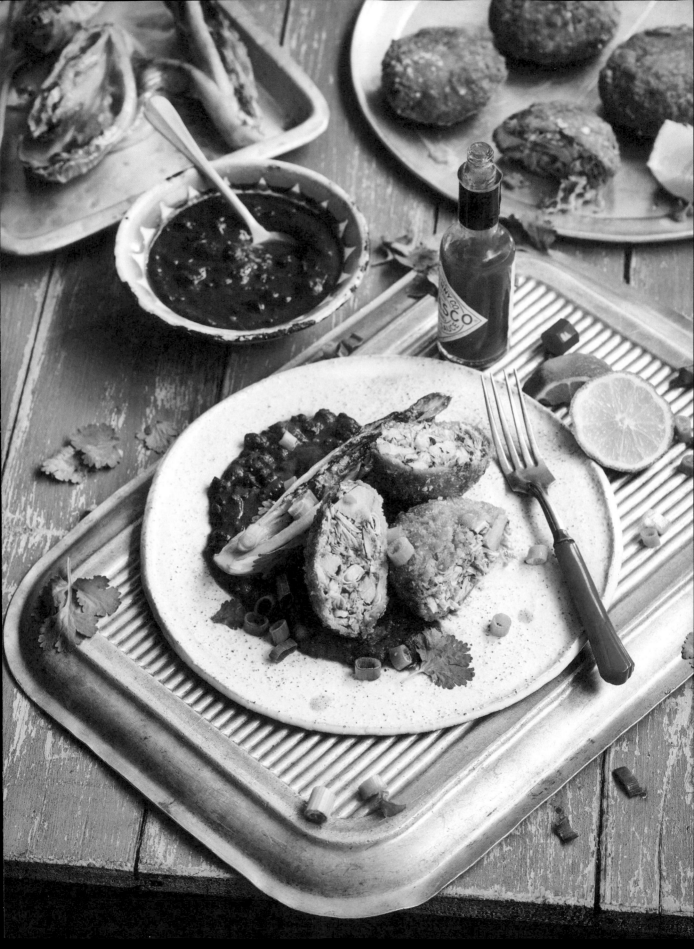

Dust your hands with a little flour, pick up around 3 tablespoons of the jackfruit mixture and form into a rough patty shape, then place onto your lined baking sheet. Repeat with the remaining mixture. Place the sheet into the freezer for 15 minutes.

Meanwhile, to prepare the coating, place the breadcrumbs into one bowl and the chickpea (gram) flour into another with the paprika and thyme. Whisk enough water into the gram flour bowl to make a beaten-egg consistency.

Remove the patties from the freezer and dip each one first into the gram flour mixture, then into the breadcrumbs. Make sure they are really well coated, you can always double dip if you like. (This technique is called pané.) Once you've coated all of the patties, pop them into the fridge until you're ready to cook them (or freeze for up to 3 months).

To make the ancho sauce, place a non-stick pan over a medium heat. When the pan is hot add the ancho chillies to toast for a couple of minutes. When you start to smell them, they are ready. Place the chillies into a blender with the onion, garlic, vegetable stock, thyme, spices, sugar and salt. Blitz until completely smooth.

Pass the sauce through a fine sieve into a small saucepan and add the black beans and chocolate. Place the pan over a low heat. Let the sauce simmer away for 20 minutes. As they cook, crush the black beans slightly with a potato masher. Check for seasoning.

Remove the jackfruit cakes from the fridge. While the sauce is cooking, place a non-stick pan over a medium heat and add a little oil. When the pan is hot, fry the cakes, in batches, for 2–3 minutes on each side. Once golden, place back onto the baking sheet. Place the tray into your oven for 15 minutes to cook the jackfruit through to the centre.

To serve, spoon generous amounts of the ancho sauce onto your plates and top with a couple of jackfruit cakes. I served mine with Grilled Baby Gem Lettuce in Orange Sauce.

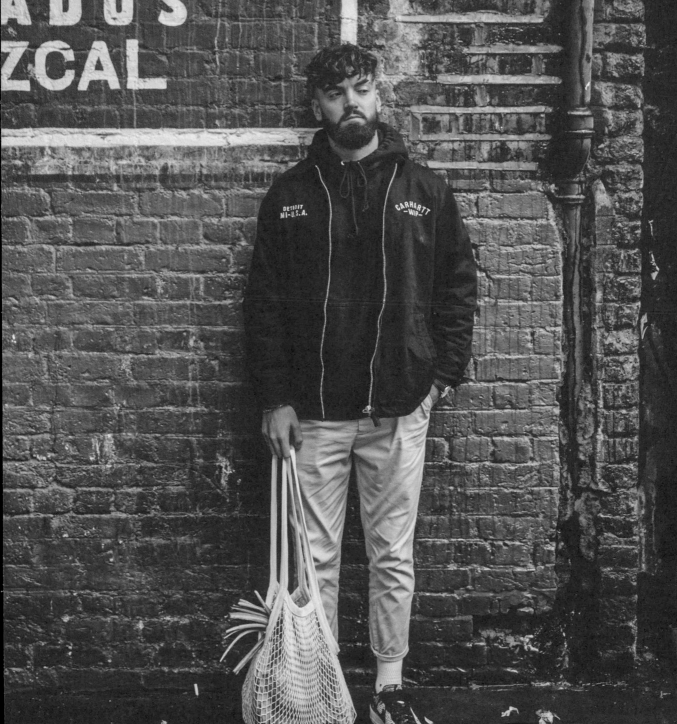

SIMPLE SPANISH ONE-POT STEW

SERVES **4**	COOKS IN **45 MINS**	DIFFICULTY **5/10**

vegetable oil, for frying

2 red onions, roughly chopped

3 garlic cloves, minced

2 celery sticks, roughly chopped

1 red (bell) pepper, diced

4 tbsp smoked sweet paprika

1 tsp cayenne pepper

2 Maris Piper potatoes, cubed

½ head of cauliflower, cut into florets

1 lemon

1 bay leaf

300g (1½ cups) split red lentils, rinsed

2 x 400-g (14-oz) cans chopped tomatoes

240ml (1 cup) vegetable stock

1 tsp sea salt

1 tsp cracked black pepper

to garnish

vegan sour cream

fresh chopped parsley

Place a large saucepan over a low heat and add a touch of oil (or water). When hot, add the onions, garlic, celery, red (bell) pepper, paprika and cayenne pepper. Sauté the mixture for a couple of minutes. I like to get the spices in nice and early so they are able to roast at the bottom of the pan.

Add the potatoes and cauliflower, then pop the lid on. Allow everything to cook for a good 10 minutes, stirring every now and then to make sure nothing is burning. Leaving the lid on is going to create some lovely steam, helping everything cook perfectly.

When the potato has softened, cut the lemon in half, squeeze in the juice and then simply throw in the halves. Don't worry, I don't expect you to eat it, but while the stew is cooking it's going to release its lovely flavour – you can remove before serving. Add the bay leaf, lentils, chopped tomatoes and stock and give everything a good stir.

Season with a little salt and pepper, then pop the lid back on and let the stew cook away for 20–25 minutes, making sure you stir every couple of minutes.

Once the sauce has thickened and it smells beautiful, serve it up. I serve mine with some vegan sour cream and fresh chopped parsley.

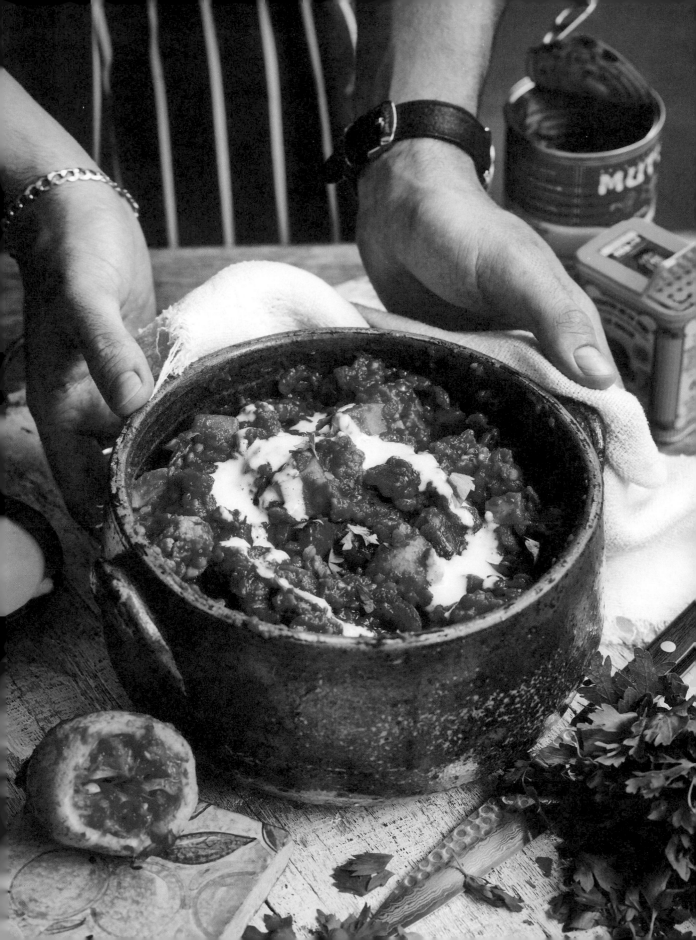

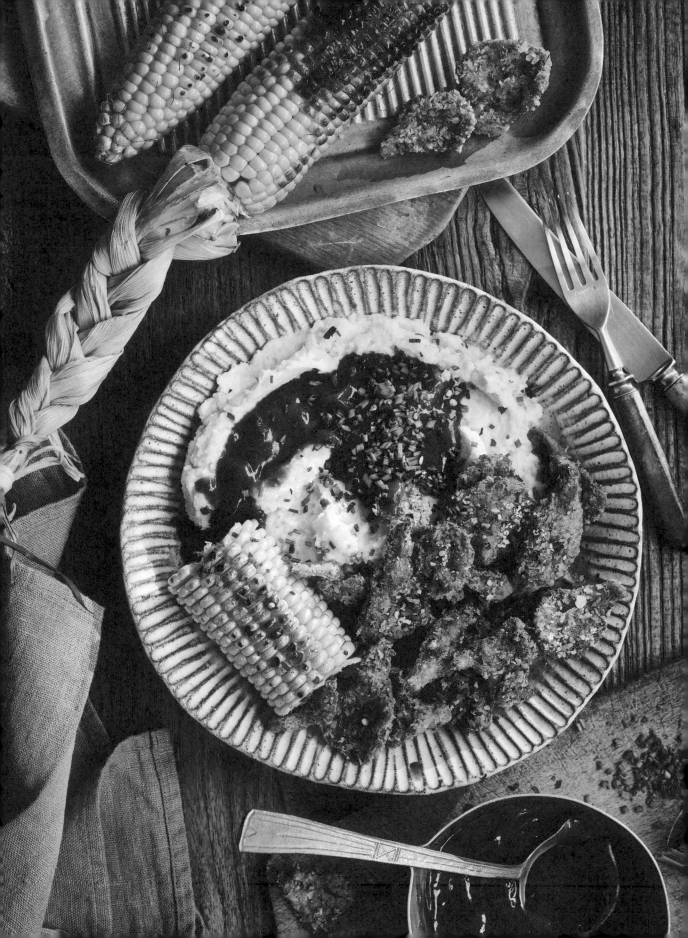

CRISPY SOUTHERN-STYLE SHROOMS

| SERVES **4** | COOKS IN **60 MINS** | DIFFICULTY **5/10** |

CAN BE GF

240ml (1 cup) soy milk

250g (9oz) oyster (pearl) mushrooms

1 litre (1¾ pints) vegetable oil, for frying

sea salt, for sprinkling

for the Kentucky coating

130g (1 cup) plain (all-purpose) flour or gluten-free flour

50g (1 cup) panko breadcrumbs

1 tsp sea salt

2 tsp cracked black pepper

2 tsp cayenne pepper

1 tsp dried oregano

2 tsp smoked paprika

2 tsp garlic granules

1 tsp dried sage

1 tsp dried thyme

1 tsp ground allspice

serve with

handful of fresh chives, finely chopped

Creamy Mash (page 170)

Gravy (page 180)

Charred Corn (page 183)

Put the soy milk into a small bowl. Put all the Kentucky coating ingredients into a separate large bowl and mix well. Dip each mushroom first in the milk, then into the Kentucky coating. I repeat this twice so the mushrooms are really well coated.

Place your coated mushrooms on a plate and put them in the freezer for 15 minutes to firm up slightly until you're ready to fry.

Half-fill a large saucepan with the vegetable oil and place over a medium heat, making sure the oil reaches no more than half way up the side of the pan. Alternatively, use a deep-fat fryer set to around 180°C (350°F). If using a saucepan, check the oil is hot enough by dipping in a wooden spoon in; if bubbles form around the wood then your oil is ready.

Remove the mushrooms from the freezer and carefully lower a few of them into the oil. Fry each batch for around 4–5 minutes. Do not add too many as you will overcrowd the pan, lowering the temperature and raising the level of the oil.

Once the mushrooms are golden and crispy, remove them from the oil using a spider or slotted spoon and place them onto a plate lined with kitchen paper. Season with a touch of sea salt to keep them crisp. Serve the shrooms with mash, gravy, charred corn and a sprinkling of fresh chives.

If you want to avoid using oil, place the mushrooms on a baking sheet lined with greaseproof paper and bake them for 25 minutes in your oven at 180°C (350°F), instead of frying.

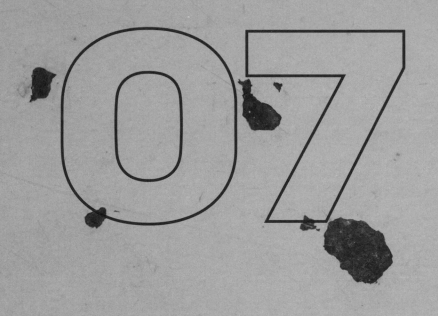

Big Bakes

BIG
BAKES

MY DAD'S POTATO CHILLI BAKE

My dad's go-to vegan bake really reminds me of home and my family – I had to include it. It's a protein-packed dish that can also be served for meal prep.

SERVES **4**	COOKS IN **90 MINS**	DIFFICULTY **5/10**

1 tbsp olive oil

1 red onion, finely chopped

4 garlic cloves, minced

2 carrots, finely chopped

1 green chilli, finely chopped

2 tsp ground cumin

1 tsp ground cinnamon

1 tsp paprika

2 tsp oregano

2 tsp sea salt

1 tsp cracked black pepper

2 tbsp tomato purée

1 x 400-g (14-oz) can chopped tomatoes

240ml (1 cup) vegetable stock

1 x 400-g (14-oz) can cannellini beans, drained and rinsed

1 x 400-g (14-oz) can red kidney beans, drained and rinsed

1 medium Maris Piper potatoes, sliced into very thin discs

1 courgette (zucchini), thinly sliced

3 tomatoes, thinly sliced

to serve

steamed greens

Place a large flameproof casserole dish over a medium heat and add the oil. When hot, add the onion, garlic, carrot and chilli. Sweat this mixture for 3–4 minutes. Add the cumin, cinnamon, paprika, oregano and seasoning to the dish and cook for a couple more minutes.

Add the tomato purée, chopped tomatoes and the vegetable stock, bring the liquid to a simmer, then add the beans and give everything a good stir.

Let the chilli bubble away for 20 minutes. Meanwhile preheat your oven to 180°C (350°F).

After 20 minutes of cooking the chilli, turn the heat off.

Carefully layer the potato, courgette (zucchini) and tomato slices on top of the chilli, alternating between the three and overlapping each slice. Once you've covered the entire top of the chilli, pop the lid on the dish or cover it with foil.

Pop the chilli into the oven for 45 minutes. After 30 minutes, remove the lid or the foil.

After a total of 45 minutes in the oven, remove the chilli bake. It should be golden and the potato slices should be a little crisp on top. Serve with some lovely steamed greens.

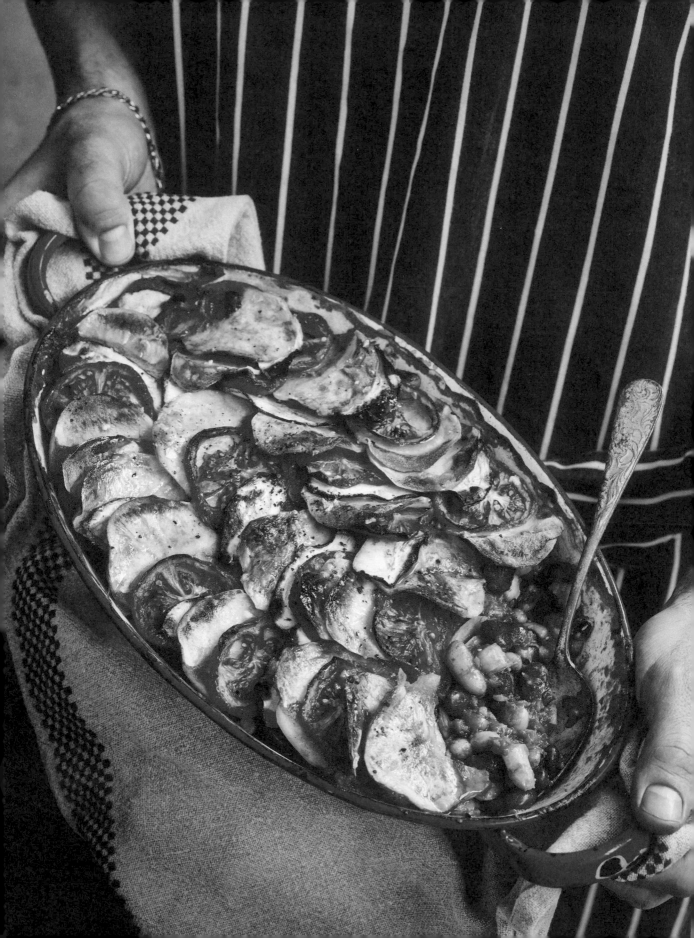

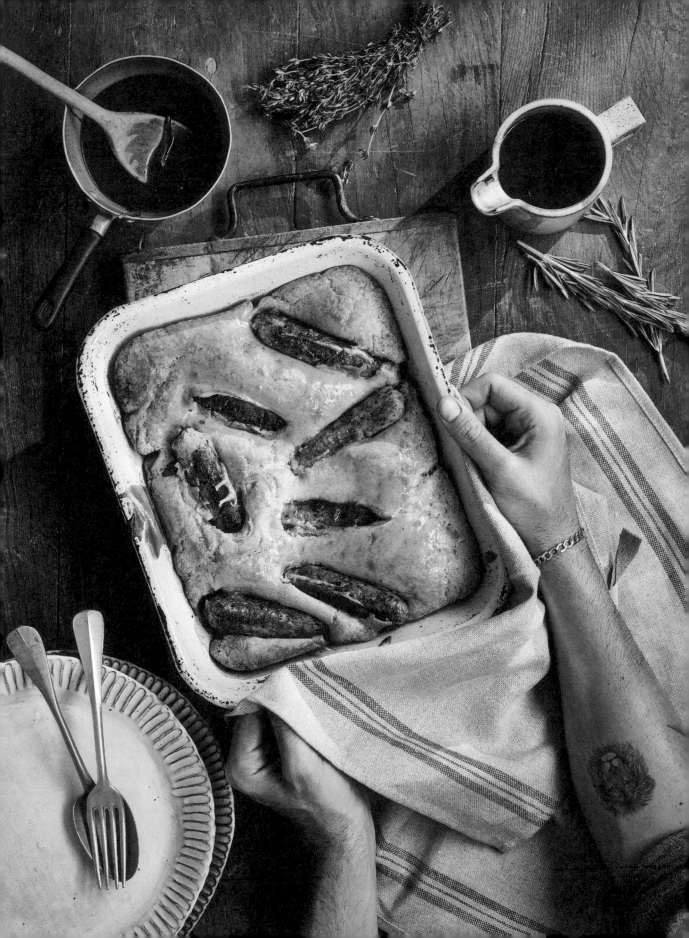

TOAD-IN-THE-HOLE WITH RED ONION GRAVY

SERVES **4–6**	COOKS IN **60 MINS**	DIFFICULTY **3/10**

8 vegan sausages

2 tbsp vegetable oil

260g (2 cups) self-raising flour

1½ tsp baking powder

1 tsp sea salt

480ml (2 cups) soy milk

for the gravy

1 tbsp olive oil

2 red onions, sliced

2 garlic cloves, minced

10 button mushrooms, halved

1 fresh thyme sprig

1 fresh rosemary sprig

1 tsp sea salt

1 tsp black pepper

2 tbsp plain (all-purpose) flour

240ml (1 cup) vegan-friendly red wine

240ml (1 cup) vegetable stock

1 tbsp Marmite or miso paste

2 tbsp balsamic vinegar

1 tbsp brown sugar

to serve

steamed greens

Preheat your oven to 210°C (410°F).

Place the sausages into a large non-stick 5cm (2in) deep baking pan, and drizzle over the oil. Bake in the oven for 15 minutes. Meanwhile, mix together the batter. Add the flour, baking powder and sea salt to a bowl, then mix well. Whisk in enough soy milk to make a pancake-batter consistency.

Remove the sausages from the oven, then carefully pour the batter into the pan. Place the pan back into the oven on the bottom shelf for 30 minutes.

Meanwhile, to make the gravy, place a large saucepan over a medium heat, then add the oil. When the pan is hot, add the onions, garlic, mushrooms, thyme, rosemary and seasoning. Sauté for 4–5 minutes, allowing the mushrooms to turn lovely and golden.

Stir in the flour and allow to cook for a couple more minutes.

Deglaze the pan with the wine and scrape all the lovely flavours off the bottom of the pan with a wooden spoon.

Add the stock, Marmite or miso, vinegar and sugar. Let the gravy simmer away for 15–20 minutes, stirring often.

Once the toad-in-the-hole has risen up and is golden and crisp, remove it from the oven.

Cut it up into slices and serve with lots of gravy and some steamed greens.

EASY MUSHROOM WELLINGTON

| SERVES **4** | COOKS IN **90 MINS** | DIFFICULTY **7/10** |

1 red onion, roughly chopped

2 celery sticks, roughly chopped

3 garlic cloves

2 tbsp olive oil

6 large flat mushrooms, such as portobello, cleaned

6 sun-dried tomatoes

2 fresh thyme sprigs

2 fresh rosemary sprigs

2 tsp sea salt

2 tsp cracked black pepper

2 tbsp tomato purée

2 tbsp plain (all-purpose) flour or gluten-free flour

120ml (½ cup) vegan-friendly red wine

2 tbsp soy sauce or tamari

120ml (½ cup) vegetable stock

2 tbsp cranberry sauce

3 tbsp plain (all-purpose) flour

1 pack ready-to-roll puff pastry

for the glaze

3 tbsp maple syrup or agave nectar

3 tbsp soy milk

3 tbsp olive oil

to serve

Gravy (page 180)

steamed greens

Add the onion, celery and garlic to a blender and blitz until finely chopped. Place a large saucepan over a medium heat and add the olive oil. When hot, add the chopped onion mixture. Sauté for 3–4 minutes or until golden.

Place the mushrooms into the pan, top-side down, and get some lovely colour on them, turning when golden. Once they have coloured and shrunk slightly, add the sun-dried tomatoes, herbs and seasoning. Sauté everything for a few more minutes. Getting a nice colour on everything at this stage is super important, just make sure nothing burns!

Stir in the tomato purée and the flour and cook for a couple of minutes before deglazing the pan with the red wine. Let the wine come to a boil before adding the soy sauce or tamari, vegetable stock and cranberry sauce. Turn the heat down to low and let it simmer away for 15–20 minutes, stirring every now and then.

After 20 minutes the sauce should be thick and luxurious. If it is still runny, leave to simmer a bit longer. Once it's nice and thick, remove from the heat and cool to room temperature (or leave in the fridge until ready to serve).

Around 90 minutes before serving, preheat your oven to 180°C (350°F) and line a baking sheet with baking paper. Mix together the glaze ingredients in a bowl and grab a pastry brush. Lightly dust your work surface with flour and roll out the pastry into a large rectangle to around 30 x 42cm (12 x 16½in).

Spoon the mushroom filling mixture down the centre third of the pastry rectangle, leaving at least a 5cm (2in) border around the edges. Make sure the mushrooms are evenly spread out. Brush the glaze over the pastry border, then neatly fold up the pastry – fold one third over the filling, then the other third over the top of that, concealing the mushroom filling inside. Pinch together any joins to seal. Carefully turn over your Wellington and place it onto your lined baking sheet so that the joins are on the bottom.

Lightly score the pastry with the tip of a sharp knife or prick the pastry with a fork to let air out when cooking. Brush a generous amount of the glaze all over the Wellington and place it into the oven on the bottom shelf for 35 minutes.

Once the pastry is beautifully crisp and golden, remove it from the oven and serve. I love to carve my Wellington at the table. Serve with gravy and steamed greens.

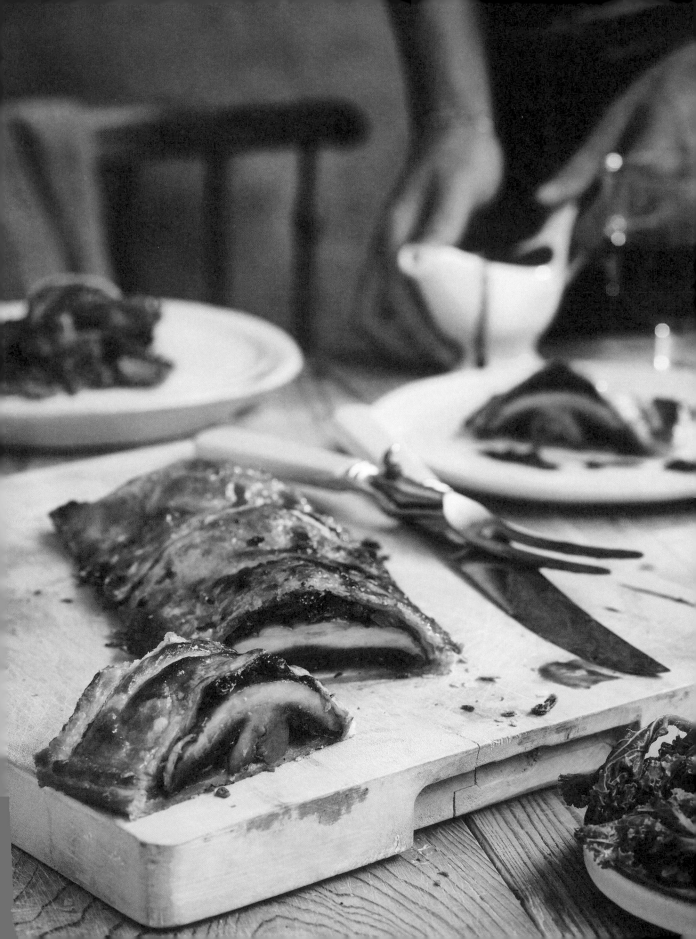

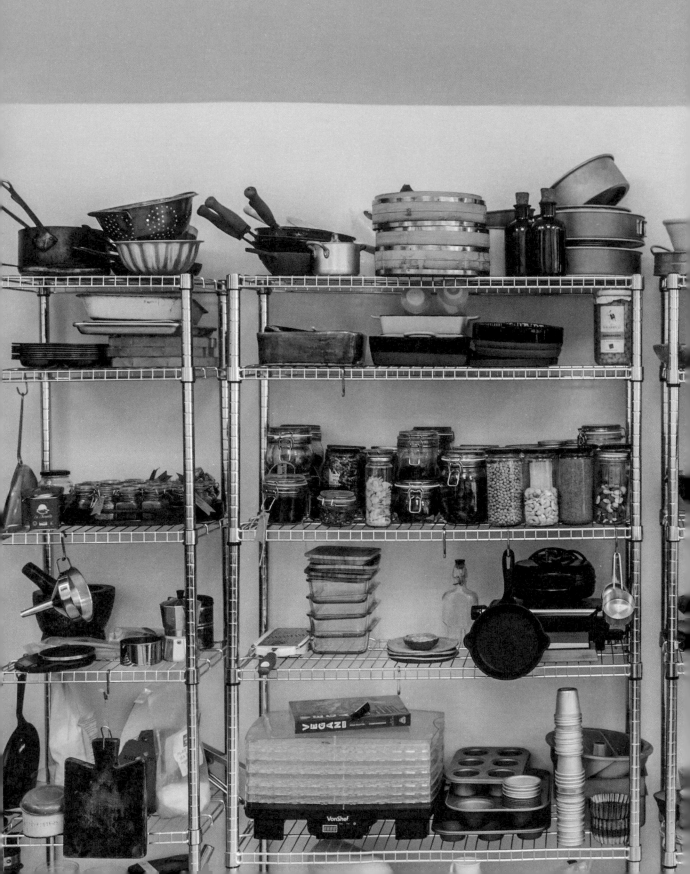

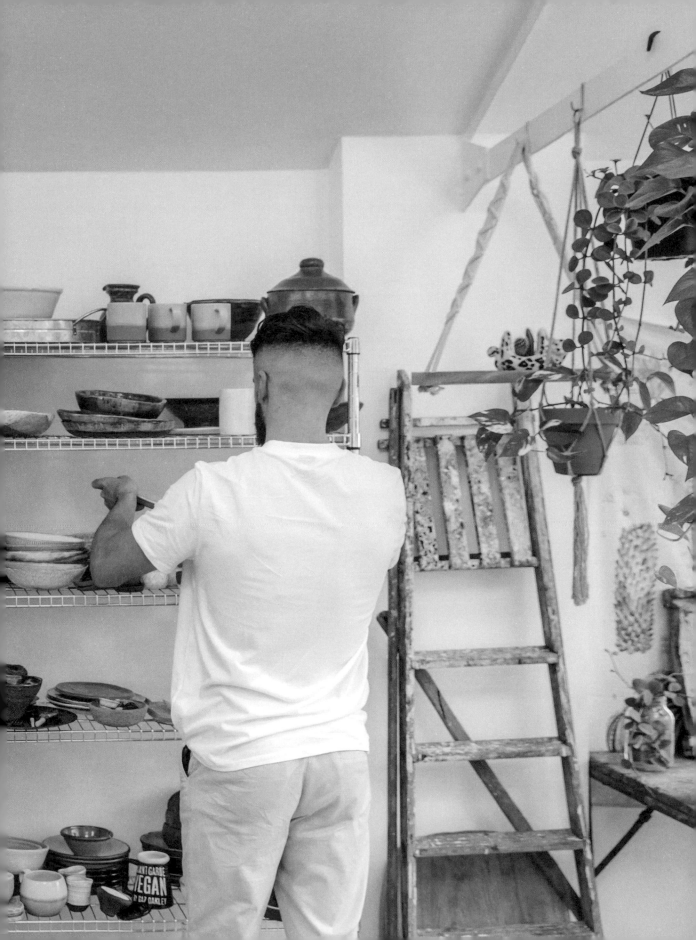

EGGPLANT PARM

| SERVES 6 | COOKS IN **120 MINS** | DIFFICULTY **7/10** |

3–4 large aubergines (eggplants)

250g (2 cups) chickpea (gram) flour

270g (2 cups) plain (all-purpose) flour or gluten-free flour

220g (2 cups) breadcrumbs, I used panko

750 ml (3 cups) vegetable oil, for frying

sea salt, for sprinkling

1 batch Béchamel Sauce (page 66)

fresh basil leaves

grated vegan cheese or vegan parmesan

for the tomato sauce

2 tbsp olive oil

2 onions, finely chopped

6 garlic cloves, minced

1 tsp sea salt

1 tsp cracked black pepper

2 x 400-g (14-oz) cans chopped tomatoes

1 tsp caster (superfine) sugar

2 tbsp white wine vinegar

to serve

steamed vegetables or salad

First up prepare the aubergines (eggplants). Trim the stems off, then cut each one lengthways into 1-cm (½-in) 'sheets'. You should be able to get 6–8 sheets from each.

Now, you need to coat them. Put the chickpea (gram) flour in a bowl and whisk in enough water to make a beaten-egg consistency. Put the flour in another bowl and the breadcrumbs in another. Dip a sheet of aubergine first in the dry flour, then the wet gram flour mixture and finally the breadcrumbs. Repeat until you've coated all the sheets.

Now for the frying. Add the vegetable oil to a deep frying pan (skillet), then place it over a medium heat. Test your oil is hot by placing a wooden spoon in the oil, if bubbles form around the spoon your oil is hot enough.

Fry 3 sheets at a time, for 2 minutes on each side. Use a spider to turn them over and to carefully remove them once fried. Place them onto a plate lined with kitchen paper to soak up any excess oil. Fry all the sheets, then sprinkle with sea salt to keep them crisp while you prepare your tomato sauce.

Place a large pan over a low heat and add the olive oil, followed by the onion and garlic. Add the seasoning and sauté for around 4 minutes. Add the chopped tomatoes, sugar and vinegar and stir well. Cover, and let the sauce bubble away for 12 minutes.

Meanwhile, make your Béchamel Sauce. Preheat your oven to 180°C (350°F).

Once the tomato sauce and béchamel are ready, build your Eggplant Parm. Take a large baking dish, ladle some tomato sauce into the bottom, then add a layer of aubergine, then a layer of fresh basil, followed by béchamel and a sprinkling of vegan cheese. Repeat the layers until you've filled your dish to the top. Make sure that the last layer is béchamel and cheese.

Bake on the middle shelf of the oven for 35 minutes. Once cooked, it should be beautiful and golden on top. Remove from the oven and let it sit for at least 10 minutes, before serving with lots of vegetables or a big salad.

To avoid using oil, place the coated aubergine sheets on a lined baking sheet and bake for 20 minutes.

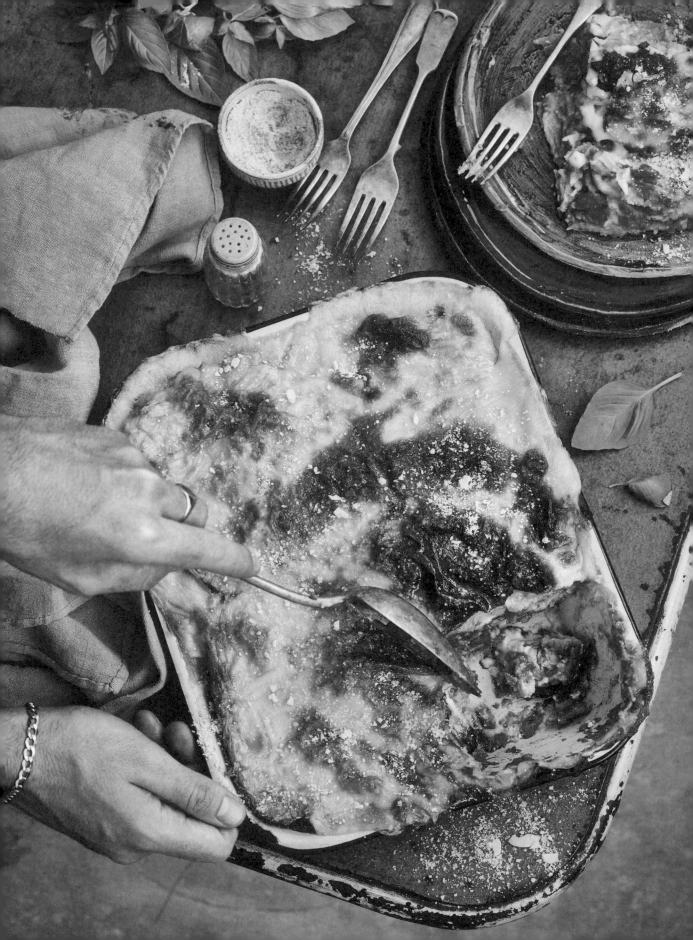

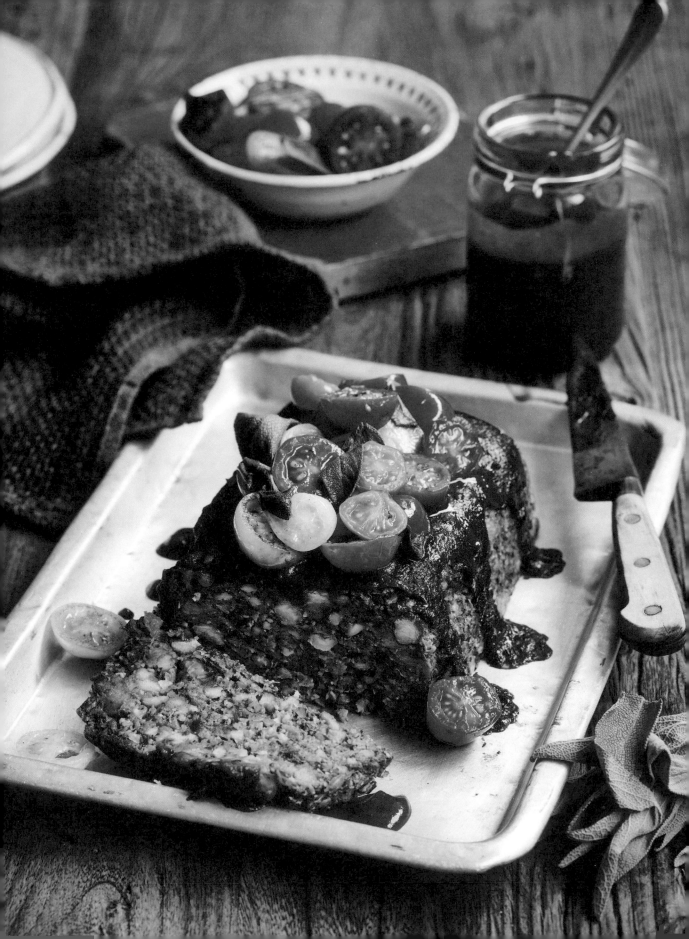

BBQ 'MEAT' LOAF

SERVES 6	COOKS IN **90 MINS**	DIFFICULTY **5/10**

150g (1½ cups) sweet potato, cubed

250g (9oz) portobello mushrooms

2 tbsp olive oil

1 onion, finely chopped

3 garlic cloves, minced

1 red (bell) pepper, diced

2 tsp dried sage

2 tsp dried rosemary

2 tsp dried thyme

1 tsp cayenne pepper

125g (1 cup) walnuts,
finely chopped

50g (1 cup) panko breadcrumbs

1 x 400-g (14-oz) can chickpeas
(garbanzos), drained

zest of 1 lemon

sea salt and black pepper

for the BBQ glaze

230g (1 cup) tomato ketchup

3 tsp English mustard

5 tbsp balsamic vinegar

1 tsp smoked paprika

1 tbsp soy sauce or tamari

3 tbsp coconut sugar

1 tbsp cumin

1 tsp garlic powder

½ tsp allspice

to garnish

handful of fresh sage, sautéed

fresh cherry tomatoes, halved

Preheat your oven to 180°C (350°F). Line a medium-sized loaf tin with greaseproof paper.

Steam the sweet potato until the flesh is soft. Add the mushrooms to a blender and blitz until they are finely chopped.

Place a large non-stick saucepan over a medium heat. Add the oil and, when hot, add the mushrooms. Sauté them for around 5 minutes so that you get rid of some of the water inside them and get them nicely golden.

Next, add the onion, garlic and red (bell) pepper to the pan, plus the herbs, spices and a pinch each of sea salt and black pepper. Sauté the mixture for a further 5 minutes, stirring often.

When you've got a nice colour on everything, add the sweet potato. Sauté the mix for a few more minutes before adding the breadcrumbs, chopped walnuts, chickpeas (garbanzos) and lemon zest. Stir until all the ingredients are well combined. Turn the heat off, then use a potato masher to lightly mash the mix, breaking down any large chunks of sweet potato and the chickpeas. Spoon the mixture into your lined loaf tin, compacting it in as much as you can. Place the 'meat' loaf on the bottom shelf of your oven and let it roast for 40 minutes.

Meanwhile, make that lovely BBQ glaze. Add all the ingredients to a small saucepan with a pinch each of salt and pepper and mix well. Place over a low heat and allow it to bubble away for around 10 minutes. Stir every now and then. Once your glaze has thickened, turn off the heat and set aside until the 'meat' loaf is cooked.

Once your 'meat' loaf has been in the oven for 40 minutes, take that baby out. Let the it stand for around 10 minutes before placing a flat baking sheet on top. Carefully, while holding the tray in place with one hand and the loaf tin with the other, turn the tray upside down so that the 'meat' loaf comes out. Lift off the loaf tin and peel off any greaseproof paper that's become stuck.

Pour lashings of the BBQ glaze over the 'meat' loaf, then place the tray back into the oven for a further 10 minutes so that the glaze caramelizes over the loaf. Serve immediately, topped with cherry tomatoes and sautéed sage leaves.

If you have a nut allergy, use pumpkin seeds in place of the walnuts.

CHEESEY STUFFED SQUASH

SERVES **4**	COOKS IN **90 MINS**	DIFFICULTY **5/10**

CAN BE GF

1 butternut squash, halved lengthwise, seeds discarded

2 tbsp vegetable oil

1 leek, finely chopped

2 garlic cloves, minced

2 tbsp finely chopped fresh sage

for the cheese sauce

750ml (3 cups) soy milk or cashew milk

½ onion

1 bay leaf

pinch nutmeg

pinch each sea salt and pepper

60g (¼ cup) vegan margarine

30g (¼ cup) plain (all-purpose) flour or gluten-free flour

½ cup (50g) grated vegan cheese (optional)

1 tbsp nutritional yeast (optional)

to serve

sprinkle of dried chilli flakes

Preheat your oven to 180°C (350°F).

Place the squash on a baking sheet and roast in the oven until softened, this should take around 40 minutes. Remove the squash from the oven, but do not turn the oven off.

Scoop out the squash flesh, leaving around 1cm (½in) of flesh around the edges. Set the flesh aside. Place the hollowed out squash halves back onto the baking sheet.

To make the sauce, place the milk into a saucepan with the onion, bay leaf, nutmeg and seasoning, then place the pan over a low heat to infuse.

Add the oil to a medium non-stick frying pan (skillet) placed over a medium heat, then sauté the leek, garlic and sage for 3–4 minutes. Remove from the heat.

In another saucepan, heat the margarine for the sauce over a low heat.

When the margarine is melted, add the flour. Mix well, using a spatula. Heat the mixture while stirring for a couple of minutes, to cook out the flour. It should have a paste-like consistency.

Gradually whisk in the infused milk, a little at a time. Once you've added all the milk, the sauce should be creamy. If you want to make it even more cheesy, add the vegan cheese and nutritional yeast.

Fold the leek mixture and some, if not all, of the reserved squash filling into the cheese sauce, then spoon the mixture into the hollowed squash halves. Bake the filled squash for 20 minutes or until beautifully golden.

Serve with a sprinkle of chilli flakes over the top.

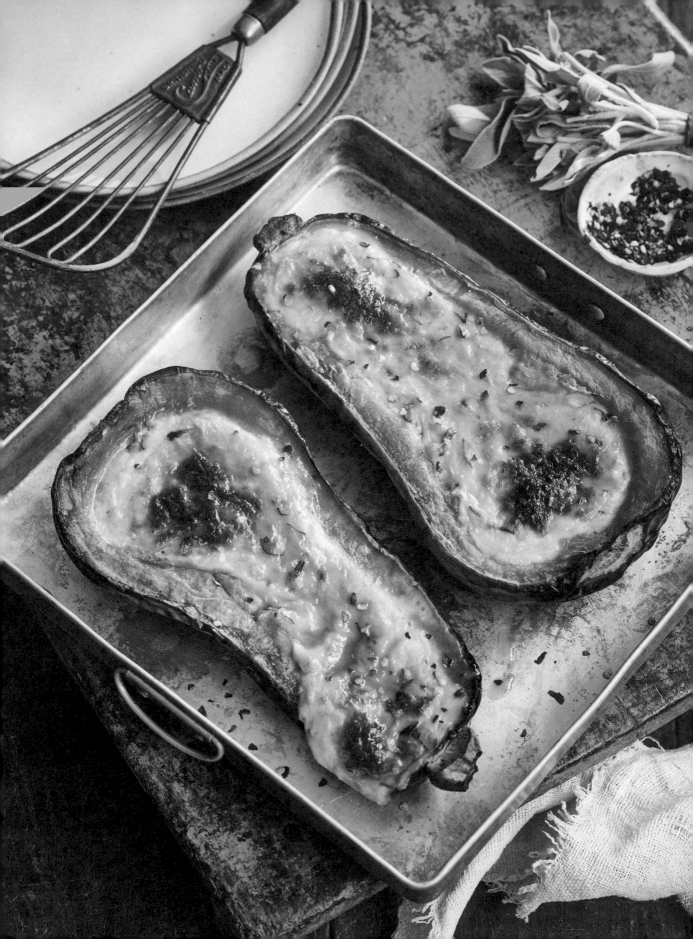

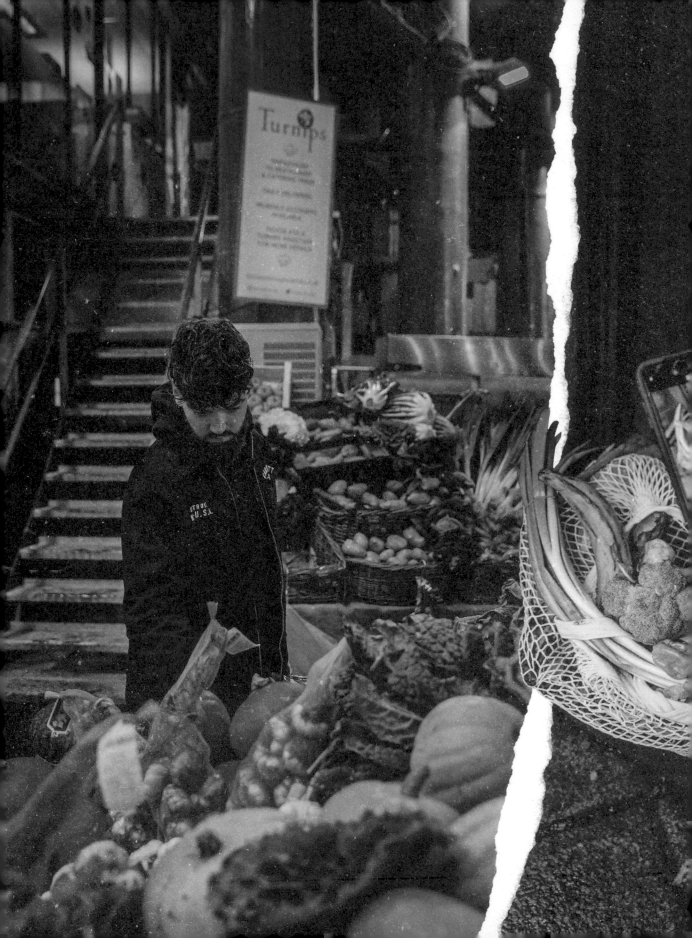

Turnips

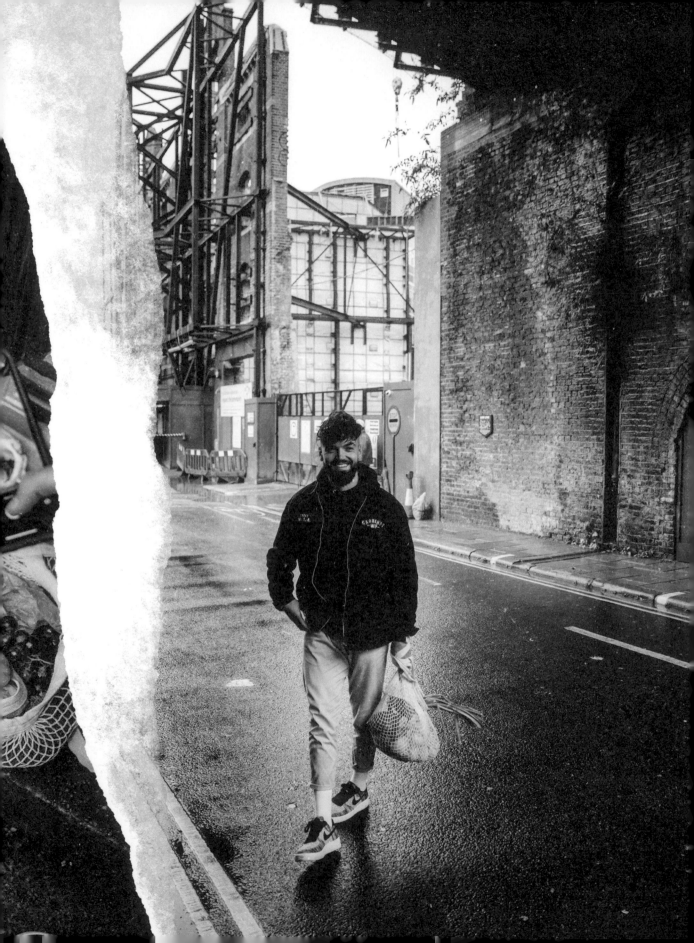

08

BURG-ERS

Burgers

BBQ BLACK BEAN BURGER

SERVES **4**	COOKS IN **45 MINS**	DIFFICULTY **5/10**

PRO TEIN   GF   MEAL ☆ PREP

5 spring onions (scallions), roughly chopped

1 red (bell) pepper, roughly chopped

8 shiitake mushrooms, roughly chopped

olive oil, for frying

1 x 400-g (14-oz) can chickpeas (garbanzos), drained and rinsed

1 x 400-g (14-oz) can black beans, drained and rinsed

3 tbsp shelled hemp seeds (optional)

handful of chopped fresh coriander (cilantro)

3 tbsp BBQ sauce

zest and juice of 1 lime

2 tsp sea salt

2 tsp black pepper

5 tbsp buckwheat flour, plus extra for dusting

to garnish

4 toasted burger buns

lettuce

Fried Plantains (page 169)

cress

tomatoes

BBQ sauce

crispy fried onions

Preheat your oven to 180°C (350°F) and line a baking sheet with greaseproof paper.

Add the spring onions (scallions), red (bell) pepper and mushrooms to your blender, then blitz until everything is finely chopped. Alternatively, you can just finely chop everything by hand.

Heat a large non-stick frying pan (skillet) over a low heat, add a little oil, then when hot, add the chopped vegetable mixture. Sauté everything for 2–3 minutes, or until softened.

Meanwhile, put the drained chickpeas (garbanzos) and black beans into a mixing bowl and give them a pat dry with kitchen paper as best as you can. Add the chickpeas and beans to the blender with the sautéed vegetable mixture, as well as the hemp seeds, coriander (cilantro), BBQ sauce, lime zest and juice and seasoning.

IMPORTANT! Pulse the blender no more than 3 times, if you overblend you will turn the mixture into a purée, resulting in mushy burgers.

Once pulsed, put the mixture into a mixing bowl and add the flour. Using your hands, lightly work the mixture together. Again, if you overmix you're going to have a mushy burger, so gently work it together. Add a little more flour if your mixture feels too wet; if not go ahead and form the mixture into patties. You should get about 4 burgers. Lightly flour your hands in-between forming each burger.

Once you've formed your burgers, place them onto the lined baking sheet. You can bake them immediately if you like, but I prefer to get them golden in the pan first. Add a touch of oil to a non-stick pan placed over a medium heat and fry the burgers on each side for 2–3 minutes. Once coloured nicely, place the burgers back onto the tray, then bake in the oven for 15 minutes.

Prepare your garnishes while the burgers are in the oven.

Serve the burgers in a toasted bun with lettuce, Fried Plantains, cress, tomatoes, some extra BBQ sauce and crispy fried onions.

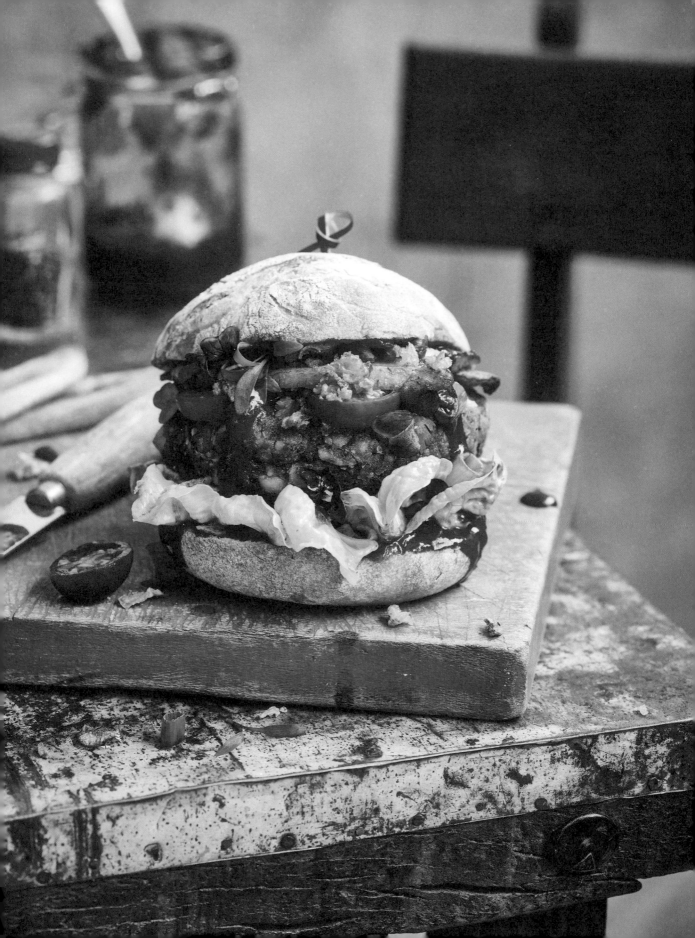

VIETNAMESE-STYLE TOFU BURGER

| SERVES **4** | COOKS IN **45 MINS** | DIFFICULTY **5/10** |

for the burgers

1 x 280-g (10-oz) block of extra-firm tofu

1 banana shallot, finely chopped

1 small red chilli, finely chopped

a handful of coriander (cilantro), chopped

1 tbsp chopped Thai basil, plus extra to garnish

1 tbsp chopped fresh mint

5 tbsp buckwheat flour

1 tbsp lemongrass paste

1 tbsp sesame seeds

1 tbsp tomato purée

3 tbsp Sriracha sauce

olive oil, for frying

to garnish

4 toasted burger buns

1 carrot, peeled into ribbons

handful of watercress

2 spring onions (scallions), finely chopped

¼ cucumber, peeled into ribbons

4 tbsp vegan mayonnaise

4 tbsp Sriracha sauce

sprinkle of sesame seeds

Preheat your oven to 180°C (350°F) and line a baking sheet with greaseproof paper.

First up, make the burgers. Add the tofu to a large mixing bowl and mash it with a potato masher until it's broken up into small pieces. Alternatively, break it up into small pieces with your hands.

Add the rest of the burger ingredients to the bowl and mix until well incorporated. Don't mash it too much as it will turn into more of a purée, resulting in a mushy burger.

Now it's time to form the mix into burger patties. Add a little flour to your hands each time to stop the mix from sticking to you. You should get 4 large burgers. Place the burgers onto the lined baking sheet.

I like to get the burgers nice and golden on the outside before baking them, so add a little oil to a non-stick pan placed over a medium heat. When hot, fry the burgers for around 3 minutes on each side, or until golden. Place the burgers back onto the tray once fried. Bake the burgers for 15 minutes.

Meanwhile, mix up the dressing (see note below), if using, and prepare your garnishes.

Once the burgers are baked, remove from the oven and build your burgers. Serve them inside a toasted bun with lots of the dressing, and the garnishes: carrot, watercress, spring onions (scallions), sesame seeds, cucumber, vegan mayonnaise and Sriracha.

Pep up your burgers by adding this hot and zingy dressing: mix 2 tbsp soy sauce with the juice and zest of 1 lime, 2 tsp Sriracha, 1 tbsp brown sugar and 1 minced garlic clove.

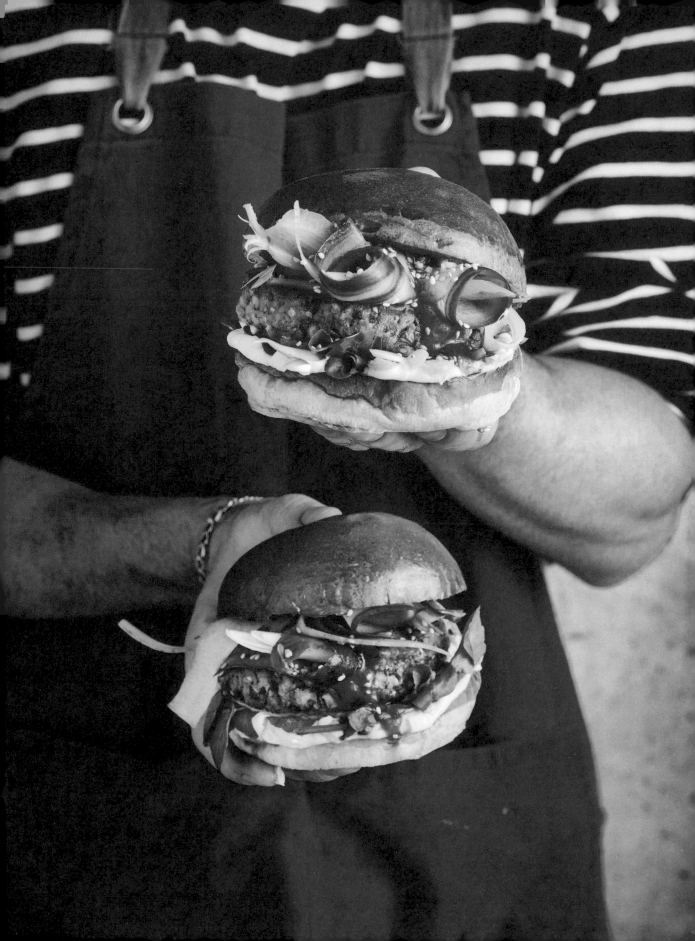

BHAJI BURGER

| SERVES **4** | COOKS IN **25 MINS** | DIFFICULTY **5/10** |

  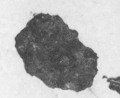

15 MIN   GF

1 large white onion, finely sliced

1 parsnip, grated

1 tsp turmeric

2 green chillies, finely chopped

handful of fresh coriander (cilantro), roughly chopped

3–4 tbsp gram (chickpea) flour

2 tsp sea salt, plus extra for sprinkling

vegetable oil, for frying

for the mint yogurt dip

1 cup vegan yogurt

2 tsp curry powder

handful of fresh mint, chopped

1 tsp curry powder

handful of fresh coriander (cilantro) stalks, chopped

pinch sea salt

for the salad

1 Baby Gem lettuce, shredded

handful of fresh coriander (cilantro) leaves

small handful of fresh mint

sprinkle of black onion seeds

juice of 1 lemon

to serve

4 toasted burger buns

mango chutney and lime pickle

To make the bhaji mixture, add the onion, parsnip, turmeric, chillies, coriander (cilantro), gram (chickpea) flour and salt to a mixing bowl with 3–4 tablespoons of water and mix well using your hands. When the mixture is sticky and comes together, it is ready.

Half-fill a saucepan with the oil and place over a medium heat. Alternatively, use a deep-fat fryer set to around 180°C (350°F). If using a saucepan, to test if the oil is hot enough, place a wooden spoon directly into the oil. If bubbles form around the wood, then your oil is hot enough.

Pick up around 2 tablespoons of the bhaji mixture and carefully lower it into the oil to deep-fry for around 2–3 minutes. You should get about 8 bhajis from this mixture. You can fry 3 or 4 of the bhajis at a time. Do not add too many as it will overcrowd the pan, lowering the temperature of the oil and raising the level.

Once the bhajis are golden and crispy, remove them from the oil using a spider or a slotted spoon and place them onto a plate lined with kitchen paper. Season with a touch of sea salt to keep them crisp.

While the bhajis are frying, mix together the dip ingredients in a small bowl.

Once you've used up all the bhaji mixture, set the bhajis aside until you're ready to serve.

Before serving, toss your salad ingredients together.

To serve, build your burgers, making sure to add lots of mango chutney, lime pickle, yogurt dip, salad and, of course, the beautiful bhajis – 2 per person.

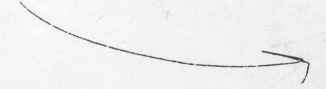

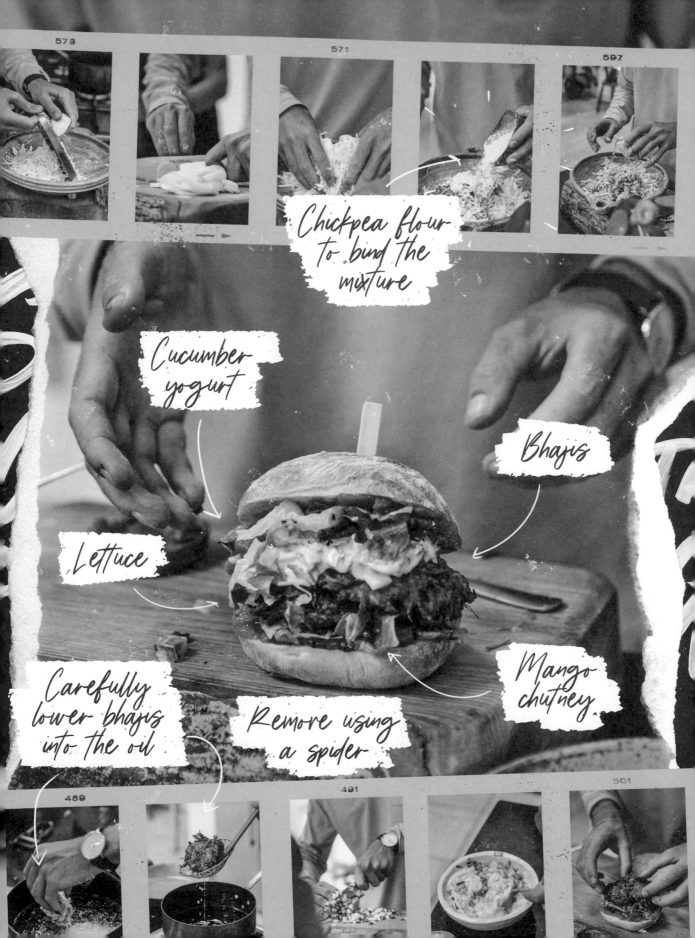

Chickpea flour to bind the mixture

Cucumber yogurt

Bhajis

Lettuce

Mango chutney

Carefully lower bhajis into the oil

Remore using a spider

573

571

597

489

491

501

SWEET POTATO PIRI PIRI BURGER

A beautiful burger that won't make you feel guilty after eating it. This is both protein- and flavour-packed, a winning combination!

SERVES 5	COOKS IN **45 MINS**	DIFFICULTY **5/10**

1 x 400-g (14-oz) can chickpeas (garbanzos), drained and rinsed

1 x 400-g (14-oz) can mixed beans, drained and rinsed

handful of fresh coriander (cilantro), chopped

1 sweet potato, cubed and steamed until soft

3 tbsp Piri Piri sauce, plus extra for serving

2 tbsp tomato purée

1 tbsp dried oregano

1 tsp dried chilli flakes

zest and juice of ½ lemon

2 tsp sea salt

5 tbsp buckwheat flour, plus a little extra for dusting

olive oil, for frying

to serve

5 toasted burger buns

handful of steamed kale

4 tbsp vegan mayonaise

handful of chopped walnuts

4 tbsp ketchup

1 beef tomato, sliced

1 red onion, sliced

1 avocado, sliced

handful of cress

Preheat your oven to 180°C (350°F) and line a baking sheet with baking paper.

First up, put the chickpeas (garbanzos) and beans into a mixing bowl and give them a pat dry with kitchen paper as best as you can.

Add the beans to a blender with all the other burger ingredients except the flour. Pulse the blender no more than 3 times; if you overblend you will turn the mixture into a purée, resulting in mushy burgers.

Once pulsed, put the mixture in to a mixing bowl and add the flour. Using your hands, lightly work the mixture together. Again, if you overmix you're going to have a mushy burger; so gently work everything together. Add a little more flour if your mixture feels too wet, if not go ahead and form the mixture into patties. You should get about 5 burgers. Lightly flour your hands in-between forming each burger.

Once you've formed your burgers, place them onto the lined baking sheet. You can bake them immediately but I like to get them golden in the pan first. Add a touch of oil to a non-stick pan placed over a medium heat and fry the burgers on each side for 2–3 minutes.

Once nicely coloured, place the burgers back onto the tray, then bake in the oven for 15 minutes.

Prepare your garnishes while the burgers are in the oven.

Serve the burgers in a toasted bun with steamed kale, vegan mayo, chopped walnuts, ketchup, sliced tomato, sliced red onion, avocado, cress and a drizzle more Piri Piri sauce.

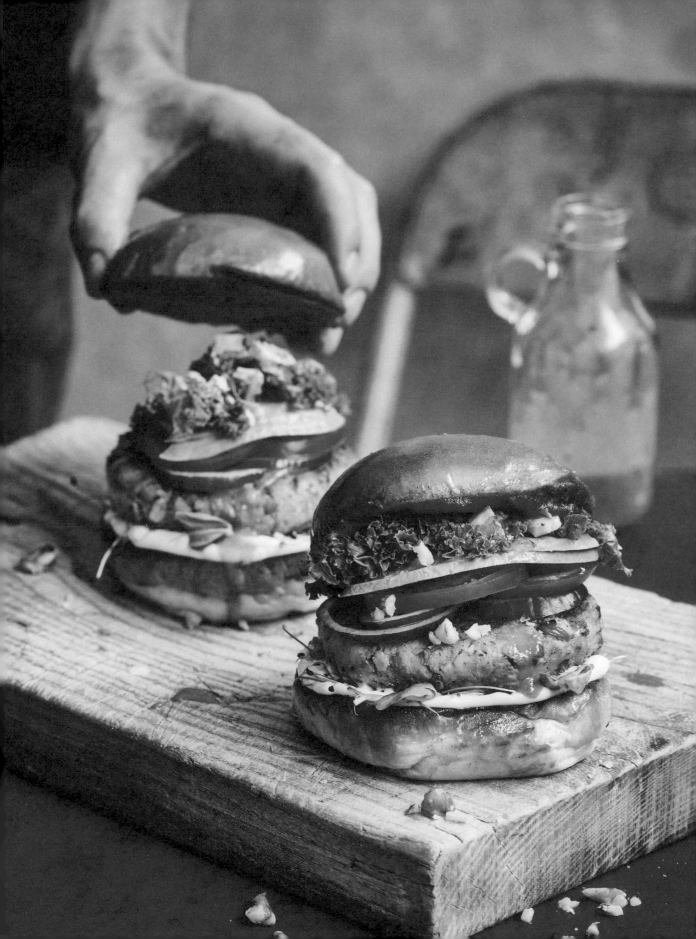

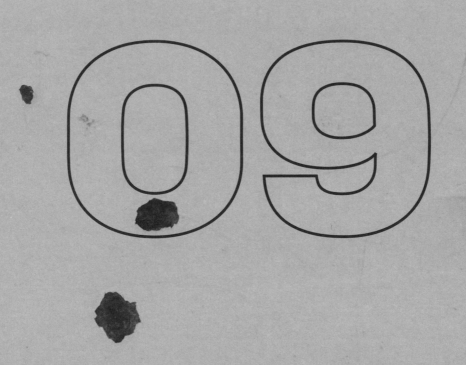

Vegetables, Sides & Salads

VEGE-
TABLES,
SIDES &
SALADS

ROAST CARROTS WITH SALSA VERDE

SERVES 4	COOKS IN 35 MINS	DIFFICULTY 3/10

20 mixed baby carrots,
scrubbed clean

1 tbsp olive oil

pinch sea salt

pinch cracked black pepper

for the salsa verde

handful of fresh parsley

handful of fresh chives

handful of fresh basil

3 garlic cloves, minced

3 tbsp capers

3 cocktail gherkins

1 tbsp mustard

3 tbsp olive oil

3 tbsp red wine vinegar

pinch sea salt

pinch cracked black pepper

Preheat your oven to 180°C (350°F).

Place the carrots onto a baking sheet and drizzle over the oil and season with salt and pepper.

Place the carrots into the oven to roast for 20 minutes.

While the carrots are cooking, add all the salsa verde ingredients to your blender and blitz until roughly chopped.

When the carrots are cooked, drizzle over lashings of salsa verde and serve.

Any leftover salsa verde can be stored in an airtight container in the fridge for up to 5 days.

The easiest way to scrub baby carrots is to use a scourer under running cold water.

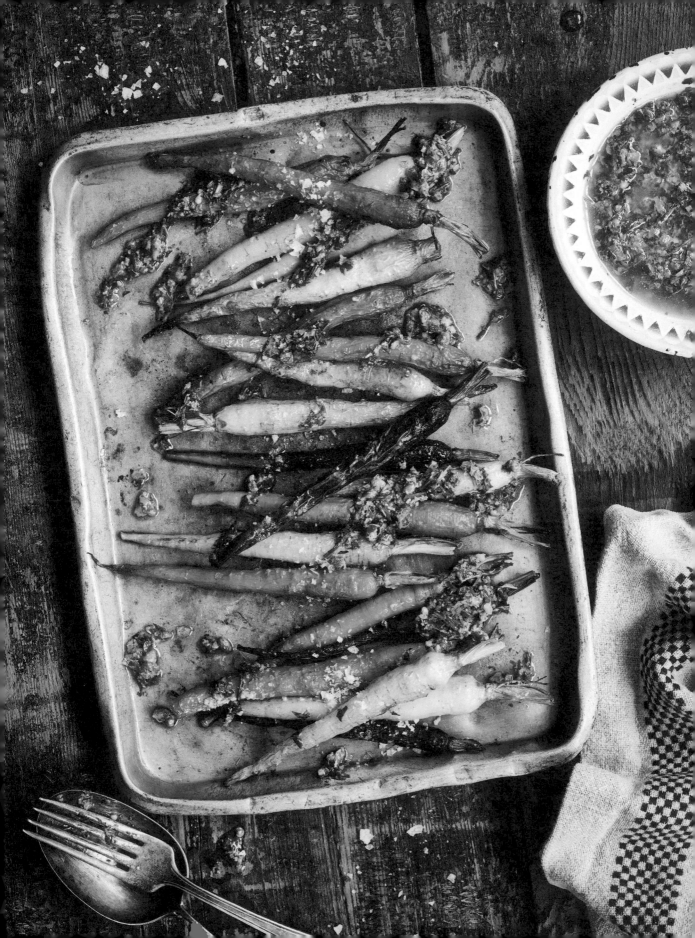

QUICK VEGETABLE COUSCOUS

SERVES **4**	COOKS IN **25 MINS**	DIFFICULTY **3/10**

olive oil, for frying

1 red onion, finely chopped

1 red (bell) pepper, diced

1 courgette (zucchini), diced

1 x 400-g (14-oz) can chickpeas (garbanzos), drained

2 tsp ground cumin

2 tsp ground coriander

2 tsp smoked paprika

1 tbsp dried thyme

1 tsp sea salt

960ml (4 cups) vegetable stock

300g (2 cups) couscous

juice of 1 lemon

Heat a little oil in a large non-stick pan or wok over a medium heat. When hot, sauté the onion, (bell) pepper, courgette (zucchini) and chickpeas (garbanzos) along with the spices, thyme and seasoning, until softened.

Add the vegetable stock and bring to a simmer. Stir in the couscous and turn off the heat.

Cover the pan to hold in the steam and leave the couscous to rehydrate until you're ready to serve (at least 5 minutes).

Just before serving, fluff up the couscous with a fork and squeeze over the lemon juice.

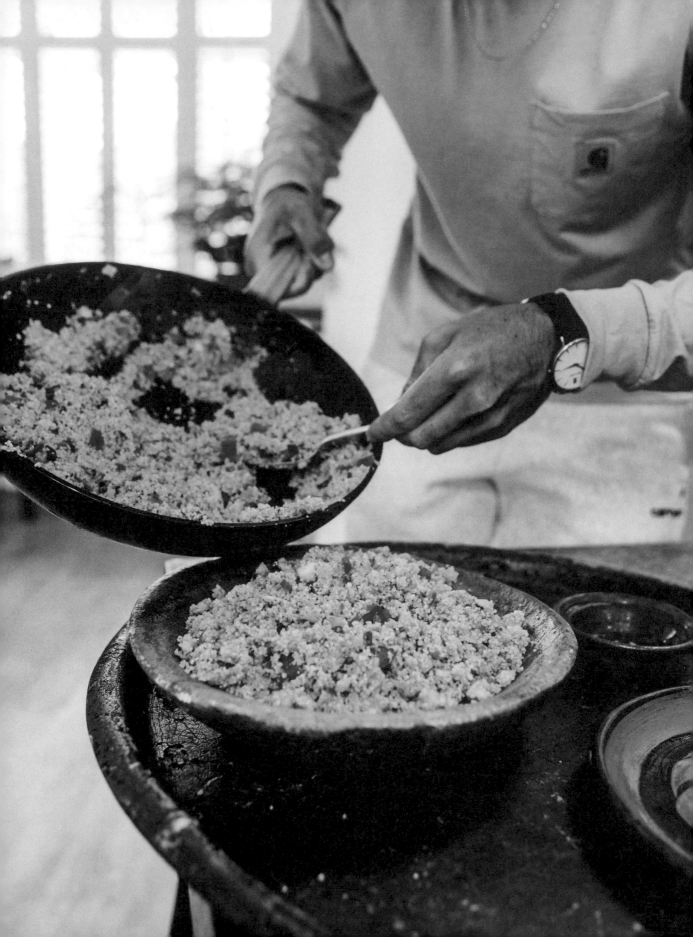

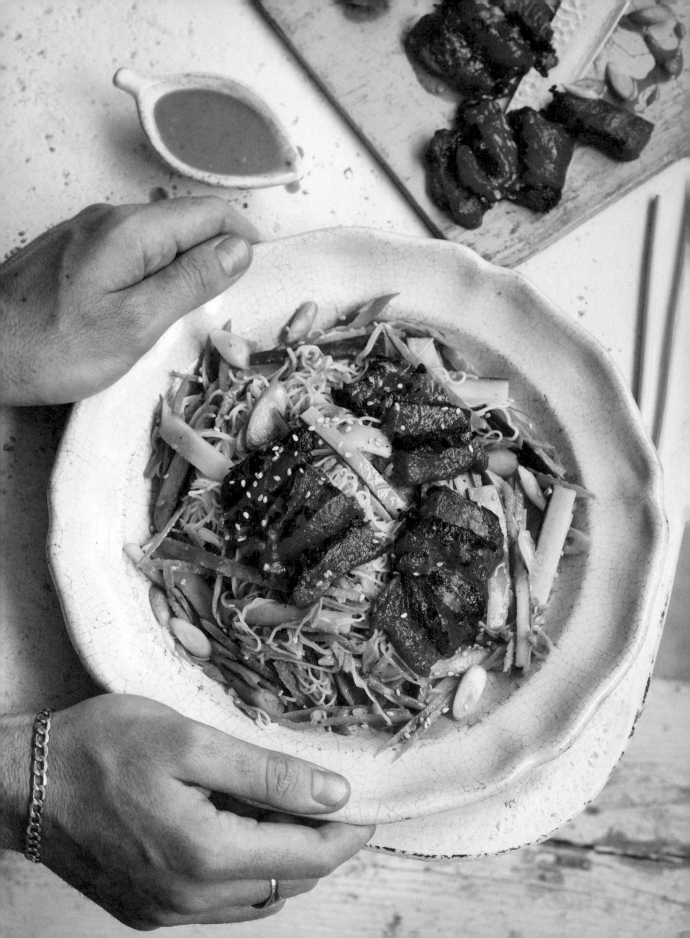

SEARED WATERMELON 'TUNA' SALAD

| SERVES **4–6** | COOKS IN **190 MINS** | DIFFICULTY **7/10** |

1 medium-sized watermelon, peeled then cut into 2.5-cm (1-in) thick steaks, approx. 6 x 4cm (2½ x 1½ in)

1 tbsp sea salt

vegetable oil, for frying

for the marinade

2 tsp tahini

6 tbsp soy sauce (or tamari for GF)

2 tbsp rice vinegar

juice ½ lime

1 tsp dried chilli flakes

1 garlic clove

1 tbsp Sriracha sauce

thumb-sized piece of fresh ginger, peeled

2 spring onions (scallions)

3 tbsp sesame oil

for the salad

½ cucumber, cut into batons

5 spring onions (scallions), finely sliced

handful of sugarsnap peas, finely sliced lengthways

300g (10½oz) rice noodles, cooked according to the packet instructions

handful of Thai basil leaves

Preheat your oven to 180°C (350°F) and line a deep baking sheet with baking paper.

Put the watermelon steaks onto the baking sheet and lightly salt. Place the watermelon into the oven for 1 hour.

Meanwhile, blitz the marinade ingredients together in a blender.

Once the watermelon is 'tender' remove it from the oven. It will shrink down and have a lovely deep red colour.

Pour the marinade over the cooked watermelon. Allow the watermelon to cool, then place into the fridge to marinate for at least 2 hours.

Remove the watermelon from the fridge. Toss the salad ingredients together, adding a few tablespoons of the watermelon marinade.

Place a non-stick frying pan (skillet) over a high heat. Add a little oil, then sear the marinated watermelon steaks for 2 minutes on each side.

Serve the watermelon, sliced, on a bed of the noodle salad.

This recipe is one of my favourites. It's the most exquisite tasting watermelon with a real texture of tuna. Make sure you get some nice caramelization on the marinated 'tuna' before serving.

CHARRED BROCCOLI, EDAMAME QUINOA SALAD

SERVES **4**	COOKS IN **20 MINS**	DIFFICULTY **3/10**

250g (2 cups) quinoa

1 tbsp sesame oil

200g (7oz) broccolini

1 red chilli, finely sliced

150g (1 cup) edamame or fresh peas

handful of toasted cashew nuts

juice of ½ lime

2 tbsp maple syrup

2 tbsp soy sauce or coconut aminos

4 tbsp mixed seeds

pinch dried chilli flakes

2 tbsp goji berries

First, cook the quinoa according to the packet instructions.

Place a griddle pan over a high heat and add the sesame oil. When hot, add the broccolini and sliced chilli.

Allow the broccolini to char for around 3–4 minutes, flipping halfway through cooking.

Meanwhile, mix together the quinoa, edamame or peas, cashew nuts, lime juice, maple syrup, soy sauce and seeds in a large serving bowl.

When the broccoli is cooked, serve the broccolini and chilli on top of the quinoa salad and add a pinch of chilli flakes and a sprinkle of goji berries.

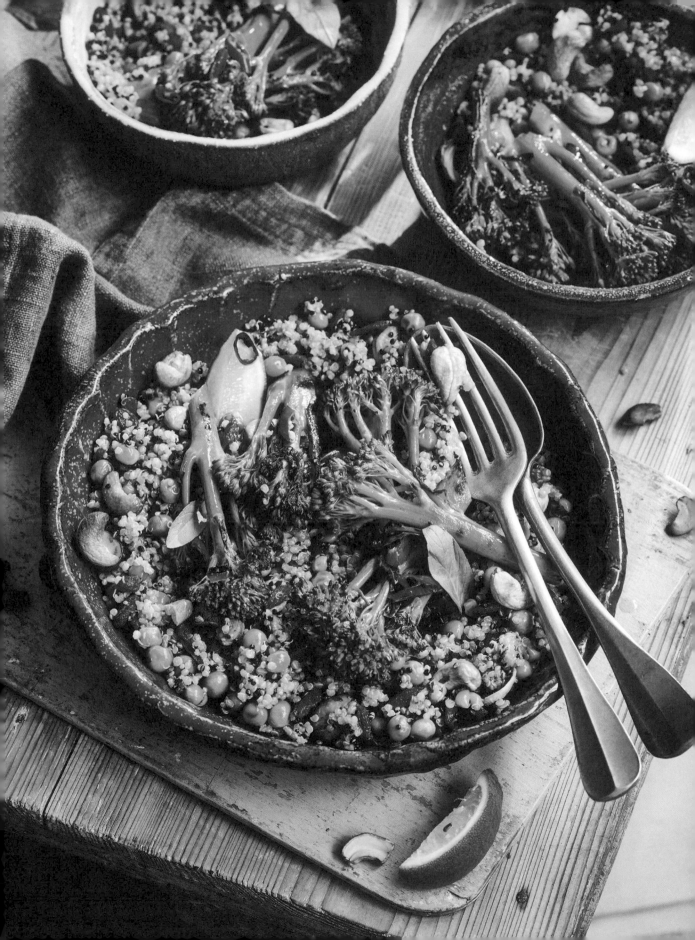

TOSTONES

These tostones – twice-fried slices of under-ripe (often green) plantain – are crunchy and delicious. They make the perfect accompaniment to my Jerk Jackfruit with Rice & Peas (page 112).

SERVES **4–6**	COOKS IN **20 MINS**	DIFFICULTY **5/10**

(GF)

2–3 under-ripe plantains

1 litre (1¾ pints) vegetable oil, for frying

salt, for sprinkling

Run the tip of your knife down the skin of the plantain lengthways, then use the cut to peel away the skin. Cut the plantain into 2-cm (¾-in) discs.

Half-fill a saucepan with the oil and place over a medium heat. Alternatively, use a deep-fat fryer set to around 180°C (350°F). If using a saucepan, to test if the oil is hot enough, place a wooden spoon directly into the oil. If bubbles form around the wood, then your oil is hot enough.

Deep-fry the plantain discs for 3–4 minutes, before removing them with a slotted spoon and placing them onto a plate lined with kitchen paper.

Individually squash each piece of fried plantain into a flat disc shape using the bottom of a glass. The plantain should be around 5mm (¼in) thick once squashed.

Fry the flattened plantain one last time, in the same oil, until super golden and crisp.

Once the pieces are nice and crispy, remove them from the oil, place onto kitchen paper once more, and season with salt.

Pictured on page 113.

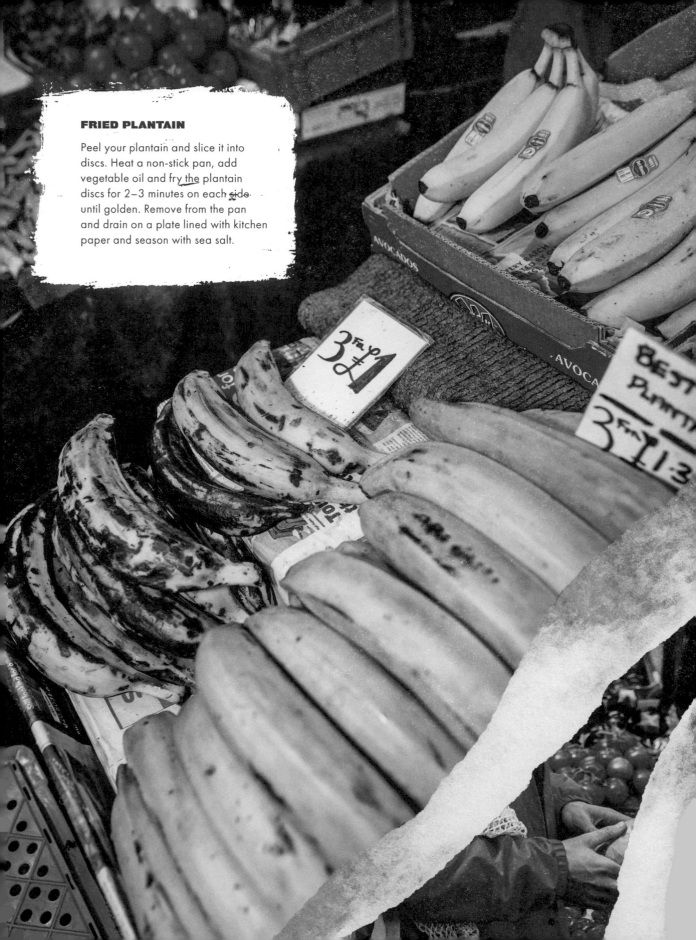

FRIED PLANTAIN

Peel your plantain and slice it into discs. Heat a non-stick pan, add vegetable oil and fry the plantain discs for 2–3 minutes on each side until golden. Remove from the pan and drain on a plate lined with kitchen paper and season with sea salt.

SLAMMIN' SLAW

| SERVES **4** | MAKES IN **15 MINS** | DIFFICULTY **3/10** |

1 apple, grated

¼ red cabbage, finely shredded

2 carrots, peeled into ribbons

½ cucumber, peeled into ribbons

1 red onion, finely sliced

juice of 1 lemon

75g (½ cup) raisins

handful of pecans or walnuts, finely chopped

handful of fresh parsley, finely chopped

Add all the ingredients to a large mixing bowl.

Toss everything together, ensuring it is thoroughly mixed.

Serve immediately.

CREAMY MASH

| SERVES **4** | COOKS IN **25 MINS** | DIFFICULTY **3/10** |

1kg (2lb 4oz) Maris Piper potatoes, cubed

240ml (1 cup) creamy non-dairy milk (such as soy, cashew, oat or pea)

½ onion

1 bay leaf

2 tsp sea salt

2 tsp ground black pepper

3 tbsp vegan margarine

Bring a large saucepan of water to a boil, then add your cubed potatoes. Cook the potatoes for around 13 minutes or until tender.

While the potatoes are cooking, heat the milk in a small saucepan with the onion, bay, seasoning and margarine. Bring the milk to a simmer, then turn off the heat.

When the potatoes are cooked, transfer them to a colander, draining away the water. Allow the potatoes dry for 2–3 minutes, then pass them through a potato ricer and back into the saucepan.

Once you've riced all the potato, strain in the infused milk. Stir the milk into the mash until it's fully incorporated. Once creamy, check the mash for seasoning then serve.

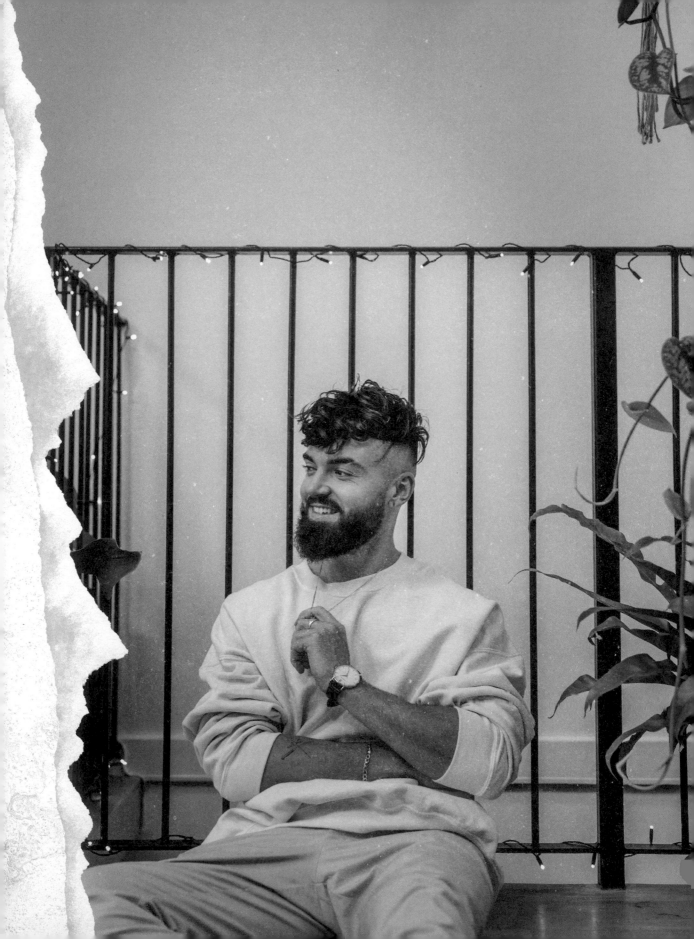

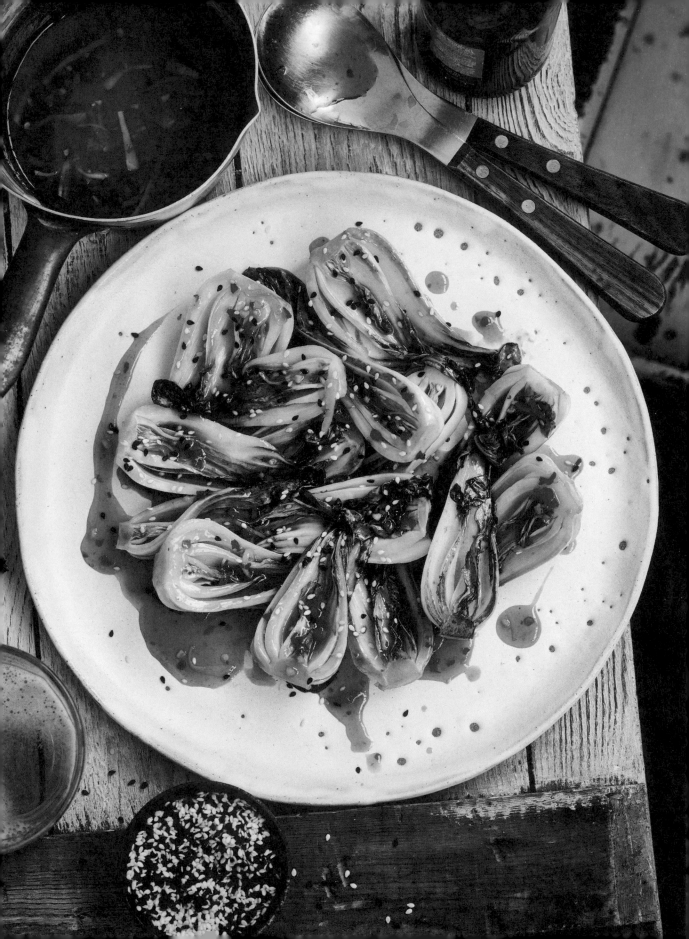

PAK CHOI WITH SESAME & SWEET CHILLI GLAZE

SERVES **4**	COOKS IN **15 MINS**	DIFFICULTY **3/10**

15 MIN   **GF**

6 baby pak choi (bok choy), halved lengthways

1 tbsp sesame oil

for the sweet chilli sauce

1 tbsp dried chilli flakes

thumb-sized piece of fresh ginger, peeled and finely sliced

4 garlic cloves, minced

240ml (1 cup) water

120ml (½ cup) rice wine vinegar

115g (½ cup) caster (superfine) sugar

2 tbsp tomato purée

2 tbsp cornflour (cornstarch), mixed with 2 tbsp water

to garnish

2 tbsp mixed sesame seeds

First up, make the sauce. Add all the ingredients except the cornflour (cornstarch) mixture to a small saucepan placed over a medium heat.

Bring the sauce to a simmer and let it bubble away for 10 minutes before whisking in the cornflour mixture to thicken it up. Turn the heat down to low while you cook your pak choi (bok choy).

Place a large wok over a high heat and add the sesame oil. When hot, throw in the pak choi, stir-fry for 3–4 minutes, then ladle in around a cup of the sweet chilli sauce.

Once the pak choi is nicely glazed, serve immediately with a sprinkling of sesame seeds.

Any leftover sauce can be stored in an airtight bottle in your fridge for up to 4 weeks.

GRILLED BABY GEM LETTUCE IN ORANGE SAUCE

Grilling is one of my favourite way to cook vegetables. It adds a great charred BBQ-style flavour to lettuce. The lovely hot citrus flavour of the orange sauce cuts through the sweetness of the lettuces and complements them so well.

SERVES **4**	COOKS IN **15 MINS**	DIFFICULTY **3/10**

15 MIN **GF**

1 tbsp olive oil

4 Baby Gem lettuces, halved

for the orange sauce

360ml (1½ cups) orange juice

thumb-sized piece of fresh ginger, peeled and finely sliced

1 red chilli, finely sliced

3 tbsp caster (superfine) sugar

Add the sauce ingredients to a small saucepan placed over a low heat. Let the sauce bubble away for around 15 minutes, stirring every now and then until it has a thick glaze-like consistency.

Meanwhile, preheat your griddle pan over a high heat and add the oil. When hot, add the lettuces, cut-side down. Grill on both sides for 2 minutes. I like to get a few charred lines on them; it adds extra flavour.

To serve, place your grilled lettuce onto a tray or platter and drizzle over plenty of the orange glaze.

Any leftover glaze can be stored in your fridge in a sealed container for up to 3 weeks.

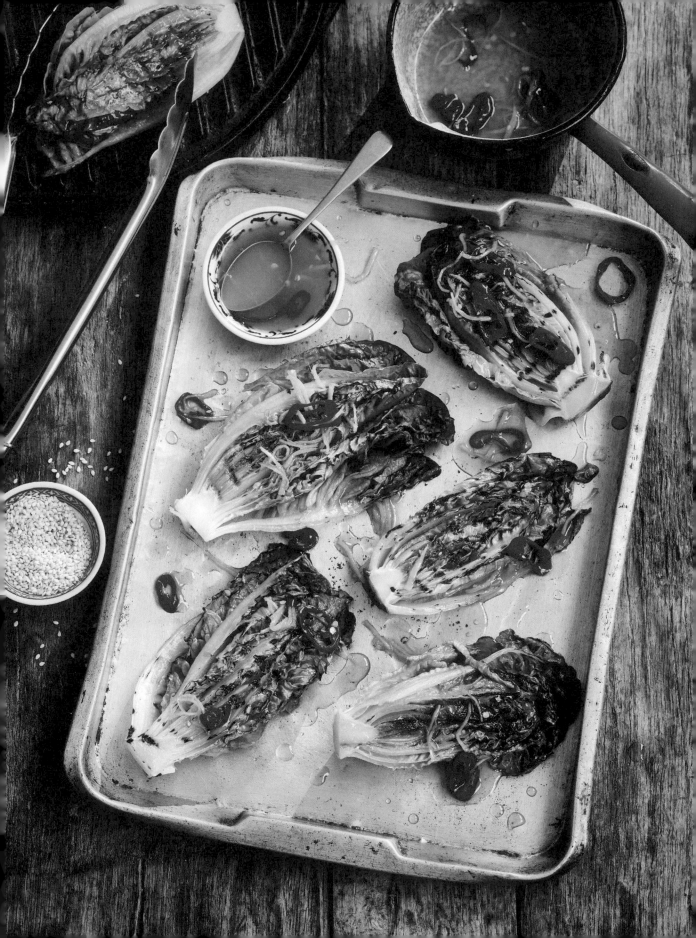

SWEET & SPICY PLANTAIN SALAD

This is my go-to salad – it has a beautiful array of sweet, spicy and tangy flavours. Plus some lovely textures from the beans, plantain, avocado and mango. It's great on its own or served as a side.

SERVES **4**	COOKS IN **15 MINS**	DIFFICULTY **3/10**

1 tbsp coconut oil

2 ripe plantains, peeled and sliced on an angle 2cm (¾ in) thick

1 tsp sea salt

½ mango, cubed

1 red onion, finely sliced

1 avocado, cubed

1 red chilli, finely sliced

handful of fresh coriander (cilantro), finely chopped

1 red (bell) pepper, deseeded and diced

1 x 400-g (14-oz) can black-eyed beans, or beans of your choice, drained and rinsed

2 tbsp mixed seeds

juice of 1 lime

2 tbsp maple syrup or agave nectar

1 tbsp soy sauce or tamari

Place a non-stick pan over a medium heat and add the coconut oil. When hot, add the plantain. Fry the slices on both sides for 2–3 minutes. Make sure you're getting the plantain beautiful caramelized.

Once fried, remove the slices from the pan and place them onto a plate lined with kitchen paper to soak up any excess oil. Season with the sea salt.

Add the fried plantain to a large bowl with all the remaining salad ingredients. Give the salad a little toss, then serve up immediately.

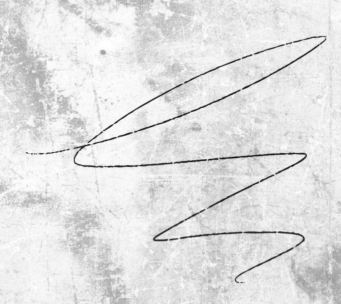

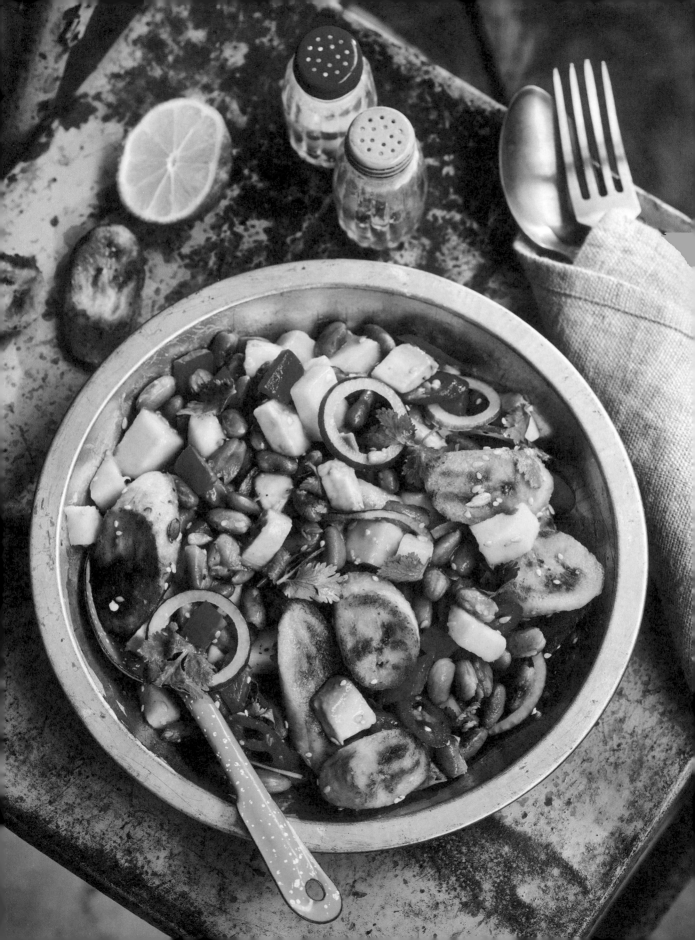

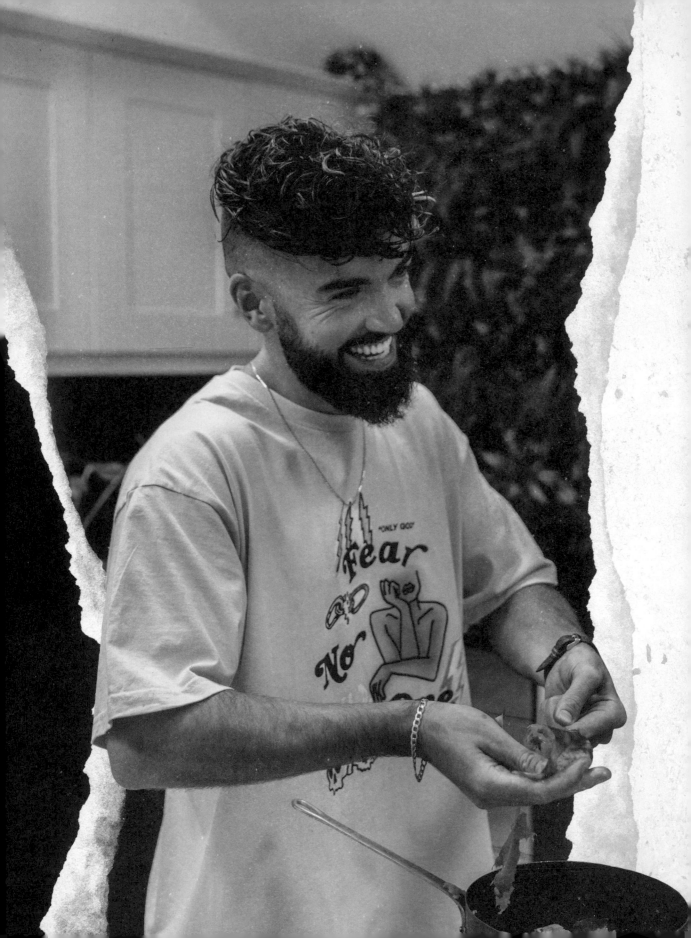

FRIES

SERVES 4–6	COOKS IN **30 MINS**	DIFFICULTY **5/10**

for the fries

1 litre (1¾ pints) vegetable oil, for frying

4 large Maris Piper potatoes, washed and cut into fries

2 tsp sea salt

1 tsp cracked black pepper

Half-fill a large saucepan with the oil and place over a medium heat. Alternatively, heat a deep-fat fryer to around 100°C (212°F). To test if the oil is hot enough, place a wooden spoon directly into the oil. If bubbles form around the wood, then your oil is hot enough.

Carefully lower the fries into the oil and deep-fry for 3–4 minutes, then remove them using a spider or a slotted spoon and place them onto a baking sheet lined with kitchen paper and set them aside for a few minutes. Remove the oil from the heat, but do not discard the oil.

Once the fries are slightly cooled, place them into the fridge, uncovered. The dry air in the fridge will remove excess moisture, resulting in crispier fries.

After at least 30 minutes in the fridge, heat your saucepan of oil once more, this time to 180°C (350°F).

Deep-fry the chips for another 3–4 minutes then remove them from the oil again and drain on kitchen paper. Allow the chips to cool once again.

Finally, before serving, fry the chips one last time until they are crisp and golden. Season with salt and pepper before serving.

POUTINE

| SERVES **4–6** | COOKS IN **60 MINS** | DIFFICULTY **7/10** |

1 batch partly-cooked Fries
(see below and page 179)

for the gravy

2 carrots, peeled

2 red onions

250g (9oz) chestnut (cremini)
mushrooms

2 garlic cloves

2 celery sticks

1 tbsp olive oil

5 sun-dried tomatoes, chopped

2 tbsp plain (all-purpose) flour

360ml (3 cups) vegetable stock

1 tbsp soy sauce

1 tbsp Marmite or miso paste

juice of 1 lemon

1 tbsp dried tarragon

2 sprigs each fresh thyme and sage

1 sprig fresh rosemary

for the cheese curds

120g (½ cup) raw cashew nuts

120ml (½ cup) filtered cold water

120ml (½ cup) cold non-dairy milk

4 tbsp tapioca starch

1 tbsp nutritional yeast

¼ tsp dried onion powder

1 tsp white miso paste

1 tsp fresh lemon juice

pinch sea salt and white pepper

¼ tsp garlic powder

First, make your fries following the method on page 179, up to the stage
where they are chilling in the fridge.

Roughly chop the carrots, onions, mushrooms, garlic and celery.

Place a large saucepan over a medium heat and add the olive oil. When hot,
add the onions and mushrooms. Sauté for 2 minutes until the mushrooms have
shrunk down. Add the rest of the chopped vegetables, the sun-dried tomatoes
and a pinch of salt and pepper, then continue to sauté for 3 minutes, stirring
often. Let the mix go golden and caramelize nicely. Make sure it doesn't burn.

Stir in the flour, then cook for 1 more minute. Deglaze the pan with the
vegetable stock, then turn the heat to low.

Add the soy sauce, Marmite or miso and lemon juice, followed by the herbs.
Leave the gravy to simmer and reduce down for 20 minutes. After that time it
should be a lot thicker.

Method continued on page 182...

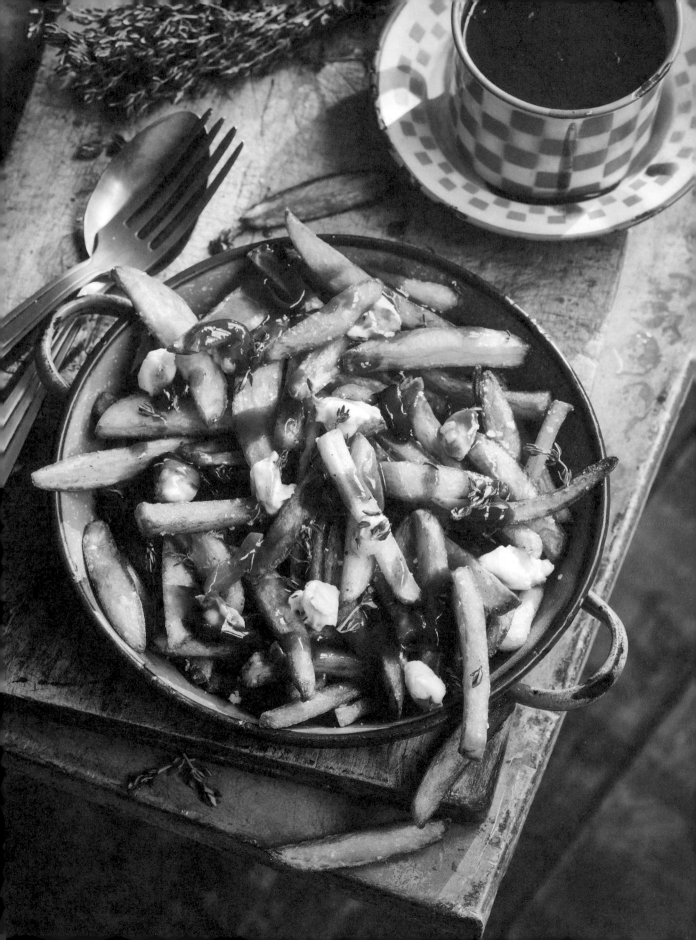

Poutine method continued...

Pass the gravy through a fine sieve into a small saucepan. Press as much of the liquid goodness out of the vegetables as possible, using the back of a ladle. You can serve the gravy immediately, however if it's still slightly thin let it reduce for a few more minutes.

The gravy can be made ahead of serving and stored in a sealed container in the fridge. Just reheat in a saucepan before serving.

To make the cheese curds, add the cashew nuts to a blender with all of the other ingredients. Blend on full speed until it's super smooth. Transfer the cheese mixture to a non-stick saucepan, placed over a low heat.

Stir the mixture constantly with a spatula for 8–10 minutes or until it is thick and cheese-like. You may need to use a whisk to get rid of any lumps. Turn off the heat once it has thickened. Pour the mixture into a container and place in the fridge to set slightly before serving.

Remove your fries from the fridge and finish cooking them, following the method on page 179.

To serve, spoon small 'curd'-like pieces on top of your fries, then pour over plenty of hot gravy. Sprinkle over a few fresh thyme leaves.

CHARRED CORN

| SERVES **4** | COOKS IN **10 MINS** | DIFFICULTY **3/10** |

4 corn on the cob

1 tbsp olive oil

For the garlic 'butter'

3 tbsp vegan margarine

1 tsp sea salt

1 tsp cracked black pepper

2 tsp garlic granules or 2 garlic cloves, minced

2 tsp dried mixed herbs

juice of ½ lemon

1 tsp dried chilli flakes

First up, add the garlic butter ingredients to a bowl and whip up until everything is fully incorporated.

Place a large non-stick pan over a high heat, making sure it is large enough for the corn to fit in, and add the oil.

Once hot, add the corn cobs a couple at a time. Char on all sides for around 5–6 minutes. Once they are charred, generously brush the garlic 'butter' over the cobs and serve immediately.

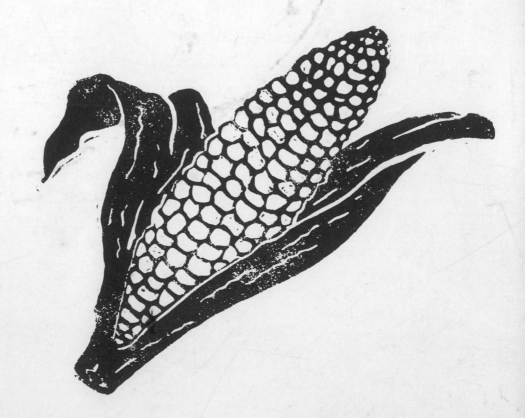

This is the most important page in the book! At every mealtime, half your plate should be filled with fruits and/or vegetables (see Plate Method, page 213). The best way to cook vegetables in my opinion is to steam them. This keeps hold of their nutrients, flavour and texture. I use a traditional bamboo steamer placed over a wok filled with water.

Vegetable	Steaming time
Spinach	30–60 seconds
Peas/edamame, from frozen	1–2 minutes
Asparagus/pak choi (bok choy)	2–3 minutes
Kale	3–4 minutes
Carrot, sliced	4–5 minutes
Broccoli/cauliflower florets	5–6 minutes
Corn on the cob	11–13 minutes
Potato, cubed	12–14 minutes
Sweet potato/squash/pumpkin, cubed	12–15 minutes
Beetroot (beets), sliced into 3-cm (1¼-in) pieces	14–16 minutes

Simply fill your wok a quarter-full with water, then place over a high heat.

Stack your bamboo steamer on top. When the water is boiling, place your vegetables into the steamer baskets.

If you're cooking something hard, such as sweet potato, make sure it goes in the bottom basket. Place the steamer lid on right away and let the steam work its magic.

If you're steaming for a long period of time, make sure you regularly top up the boiling water in the wok.

Refer to the table above for steaming times.

Check your vegetables are tender by sticking a fork into each.

A bamboo steamer is easy to clean, I just rinse mine with hot soapy water then leave to dry. It even goes in the dishwasher from time to time.

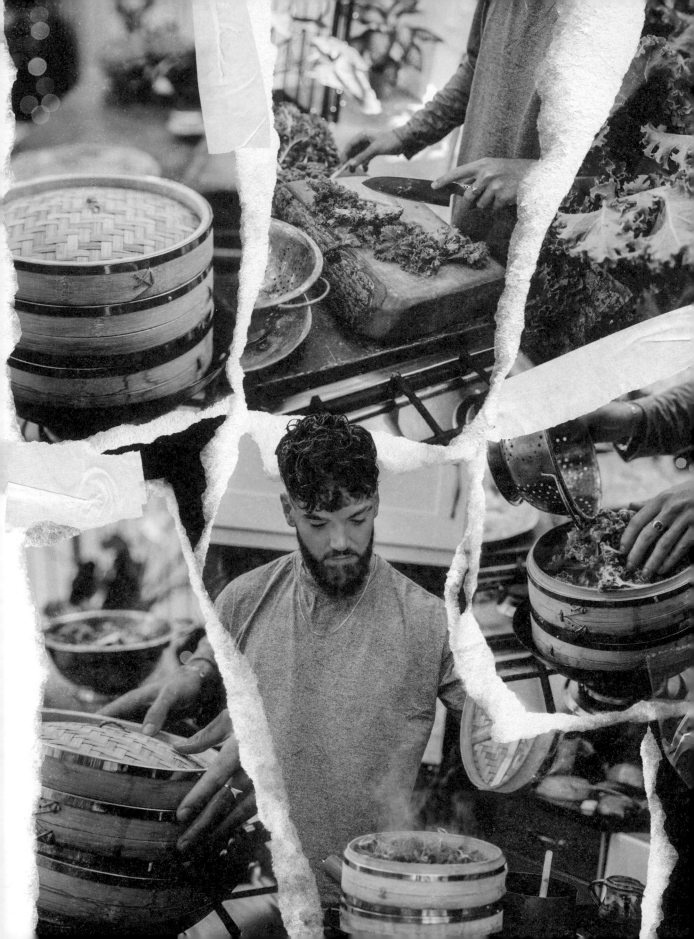

10

DESSERTS

Desserts

APPLE & BLACKBERRY PIES

These pies are simple to make, yet decadent. Feel free to be adventurous with your fillings, too – hard fruits like apples and pears work the best but you could also use mangos and peaches.

| MAKES **4** | COOKS IN **50 MINS** | DIFFICULTY **5/10** |

4 sweet apples (I used Braeburns) cut into 1-cm (½-in) cubes

200g (2 cups) blackberries

4 tbsp coconut sugar, or sweetener of your choice, plus extra for sprinkling

1 tsp ground cinnamon

pinch grated nutmeg

1 sheet ready-to-roll puff pastry

100g (¾ cup) plain (all-purpose) flour or gluten-free flour, for dusting

for the glaze

3 tbsp maple syrup

2 tbsp vegetable oil

2 tbsp non-dairy milk

to serve

vegan custard

fresh mint

maple syrup

Preheat your oven to 180°C (350°F) and line a baking sheet with baking paper.

Add the cubed apple, blackberries, sugar and spices to a saucepan and place over a low heat. Pop the lid on the pan and leave to bubble away for 12 minutes.

Meanwhile roll the pastry out on lightly floured baking paper, to around 3mm (⅛in) thick. Cut the pastry into 4 rectangles, each 13 x 7.5cm (5 x 3in).

When the apple has softened, transfer to a large bowl and allow to cool slightly.

To make the glaze, mix together the maple syrup, oil and non-dairy milk in a small bowl.

Place half of the pastry rectangles onto your lined baking sheet, a few inches apart from one another. Spoon 2–3 tbsp of the apple mixture into the centre of each rectangle, leaving a 2.5cm (1 in) border around the edge. Brush the border with your pastry glaze.

Place the remaining pastry rectangles on top of the filling, neatly sealing the edges first with your fingers. Then, using a fork, press around the edges, locking the filling inside.

Brush the pies with the glaze and sprinkle over a little sugar. Place the pies into the oven to bake for 25 minutes.

Serve the pies with custard, a drizzle of maple syrup and a little fresh mint.

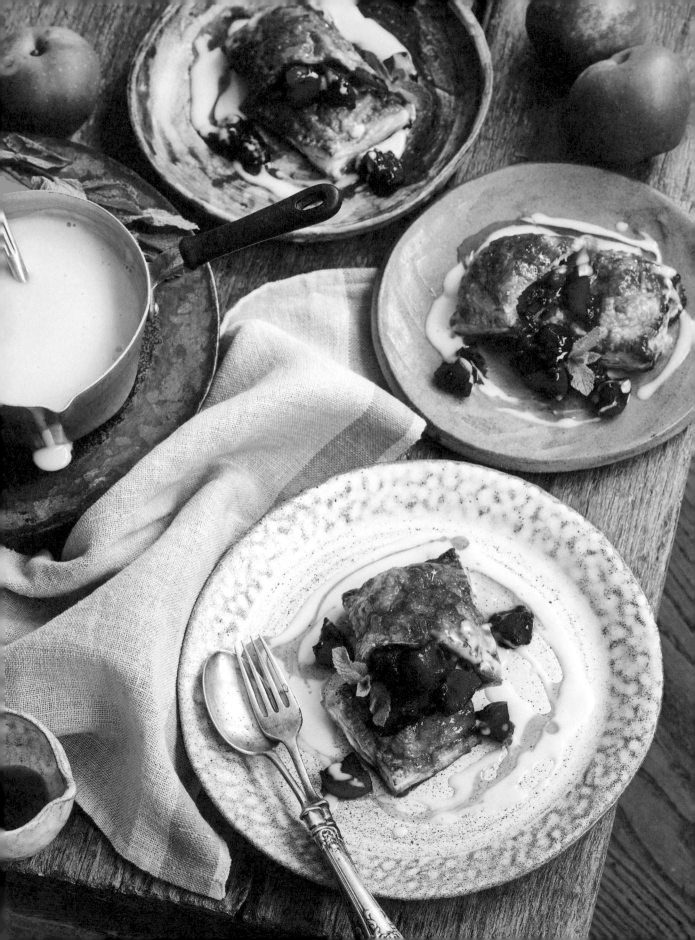

EPIC CHERRY CINNAMON ROLLS

Light, fluffy and warming, the perfect cinnamon roll recipe. I added some cherry for a slight twist – it works so well. Tear and share with your friends.

| SERVES **6–8** | COOKS IN **165 MINS** | DIFFICULTY **7/10** |

for the dough

360ml (1½ cups) soy milk

115g (½ cup) vegan margarine, plus extra for greasing

2 tsp fast-action dried yeast

475g (3⅓ cups) strong white bread flour, plus extra for dusting

75g (¾ cup) cornflour (cornstarch)

60g (½ cup) icing (confectioners') sugar

for the filling

90g (¾ cup) dried cherries

2 tbsp almond butter

1 tbsp ground cinnamon

5 tbsp maple syrup

First up, prepare your dough. Gently heat the soy milk and margarine in a saucepan over a low heat until the margarine has melted and the mixture is lukewarm. Whisk in the yeast, then set the mixture aside for 5 minutes.

Meanwhile, add the flour, cornflour (cornstarch) and icing (confectioners') sugar to a stand mixer fitted with a dough hook or a large mixing bowl. Pour in the soy milk mixture, and, if using, turn the mixer to medium speed to knead for 5–6 minutes. Otherwise, knead by hand.

Once the dough has been kneaded, lightly grease a mixing bowl with margarine and place the dough in the bowl. Cover the bowl with a clean kitchen (dish) towel and place it somewhere warm for around 1 hour to double in size. Alternatively, you can place the dough in the fridge overnight to rise slowly.

While the dough is resting, blitz together the filling ingredients, adding a little water to help it blend. Once blended, the mix should have a syrup-like consistency, with very small cherry pieces running through it.

Line a baking sheet or a circular 23-cm (9-in) cake tin with a loose bottom with greaseproof paper.

Lightly flour your work surface and turn the risen dough out of your bowl. Roll the dough into a long rectangular shape around 1cm (½in) thick.

Evenly spread the filling mixture over the dough, then roll up the dough widthways. Once rolled, cut the dough roll into 8 even-sized slices.

Arrange the pieces, cut-side up, in your lined tray. Cover the tray with a clean kitchen towel and place somewhere warm for around 45 minutes or until nicely risen.

Preheat your oven to 180°C (350°F).

for the sticky glaze

120ml (½ cup) maple syrup

175g (¾ cup) vegan margarine

handful of flaked almonds

for the icing (frosting)

120g (1 cup) icing
(confectioners') sugar

60ml (¼ cup) almond milk

1 tsp vanilla extract

To make the sticky glaze. Heat the maple syrup and margarine in a saucepan over a low heat. Once the margarine has melted, remove it from the heat.

Once the rolls have risen, pour over half of the sticky glaze.

Bake the rolls on the bottom shelf of the oven for 25 minutes before removing them from the oven to carefully add the remaining sticky glaze and some of the flaked almonds. Place the rolls back into the oven for a further 10 minutes until beautiful and golden.

Meanwhile, make the icing (frosting). Mix together the icing sugar, almond milk and vanilla.

Remove the rolls from the oven and allow to cool before removing from the tin or tray. Allow to cool completely on a wire rack, then pour over the icing, scatter with the remaining flaked almonds and serve.

Pictured on pages 192–3.

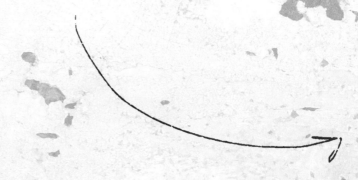

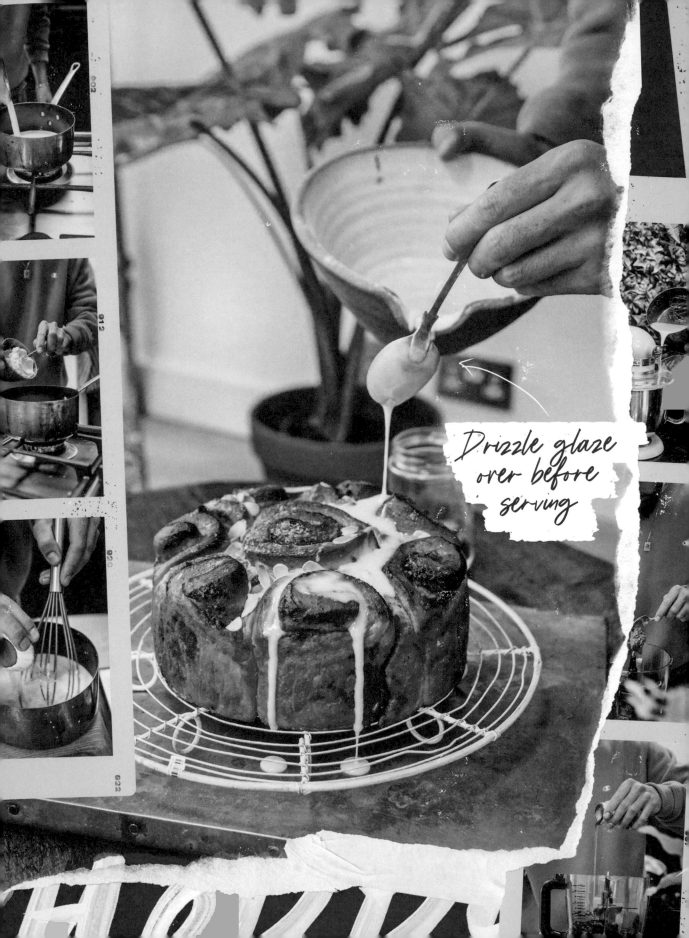

Drizzle glaze
over before
serving

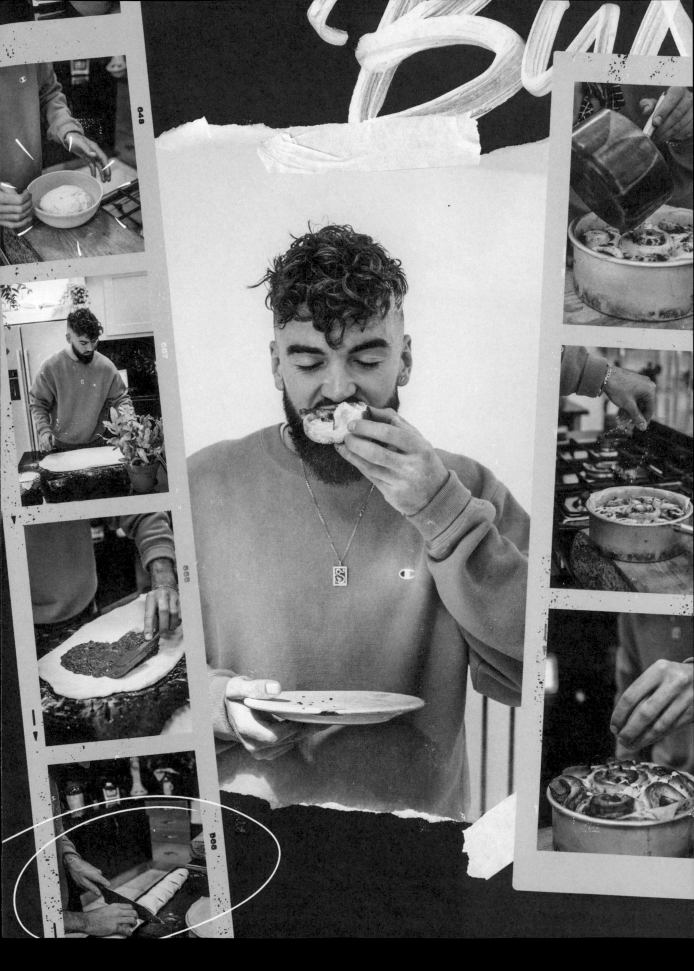

STICKY ORANGE CRÊPES

SERVES 4-6	COOKS IN 35 MINS	DIFFICULTY 3/10

for the crêpes

270g (2 cups) plain (all-purpose) flour or gluten-free flour

pinch sea salt

720ml (3 cups) non-dairy milk

vegetable oil, for frying

for the orange sauce

240ml (1 cup) orange juice

1 orange, peeled and cut into segments

230g (1 cup) caster (superfine) sugar

1 star anise

35ml (1 shot) orange liqueur

First up, prepare your crêpe batter. Add the flour and sea salt to a mixing bowl, then whisk in the non-dairy milk. Set the batter aside for 10 minutes.

Meanwhile, to make the sauce, add all the ingredients to a small saucepan and place it over a low heat. Let the sauce bubble away and thicken up for around 15 minutes, stirring occasionally.

Lightly oil a non-stick frying pan (skillet) and place over a medium heat. Add enough crêpe batter to cover the surface of the pan. Use the back of a ladle to spread the batter out, if necessary. Cook each crêpe for around 2 minutes on each side or until golden, adding more oil as needed.

Once you've used up all the batter, serve the crêpes with plenty of orange sauce drizzled over the top.

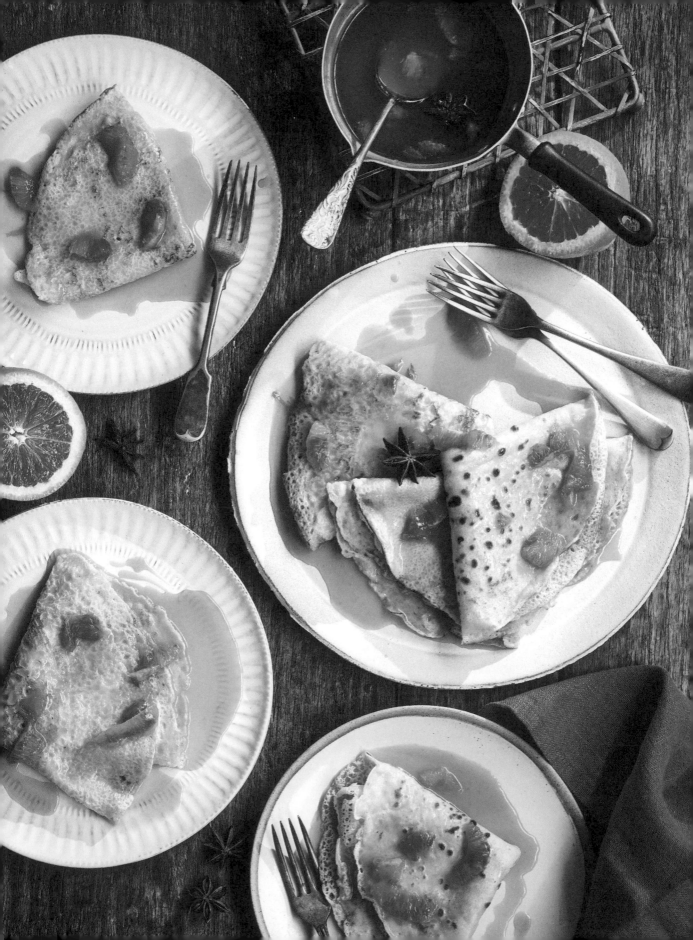

TOFFEE APPLE CHOCOLATE BROWNIE PUDDING

This tasty dessert shouts autumn/winter to me. The caramelized toffee apples just make me think of the Halloween season. They go so well with the rich, light brownie pudding.

SERVES **6–8**	COOKS IN **60 MINS**	DIFFICULTY **5/10**

CAN BE GF

200g (1½ cups) dairy-free dark chocolate

5 tbsp vegan margarine

5 tbsp caster (superfine) sugar

2 Braeburn apples, peeled and diced

170g (1½ cups) self-raising flour or gluten-free flour

180g (1¼ cups) light brown sugar

3 tbsp cocoa powder

pinch sea salt

pinch ground cinnamon

240ml (1 cup) non-dairy milk

handful of walnuts

handful of pumpkin seeds

to serve

Caramel Sauce (page 210)

Preheat your oven to 180°C (350°F) and line a 25.5-cm (10-in) square baking sheet with greaseproof paper.

Fill a small saucepan a quarter full with water, and place over a low heat. Place a heatproof bowl on top, then add the chocolate and vegan margarine to the bowl. Let the mixture melt together. If the water starts to boil, turn off the heat and let the residual heat melt the chocolate.

Meanwhile, place a non-stick frying pan (skillet) over a medium heat and add the caster (superfine) sugar. Let the sugar melt down into a caramel, swirling the pan to help it melt. Once the sugar has melted, add the apples and toss the pan to get them coated nicely. Let the apples cook down for 3–4 minutes, then turn off the heat.

Meanwhile, add the flour, light brown sugar, cocoa, salt and cinnamon to a mixing bowl, then mix well. Fold in the non-dairy milk, followed by the melted chocolate mixture.

Pour the brownie mixture into your lined baking sheet, spreading the mixture out evenly. Top the mixture with the caramelized apples, walnuts and pumpkin seeds.

Bake for 25–30 minutes, until lightly coloured on top and springy to the touch.

Once baked, let the brownie cool completely on a wire rack, then cut into slices and serve with Caramel Sauce.

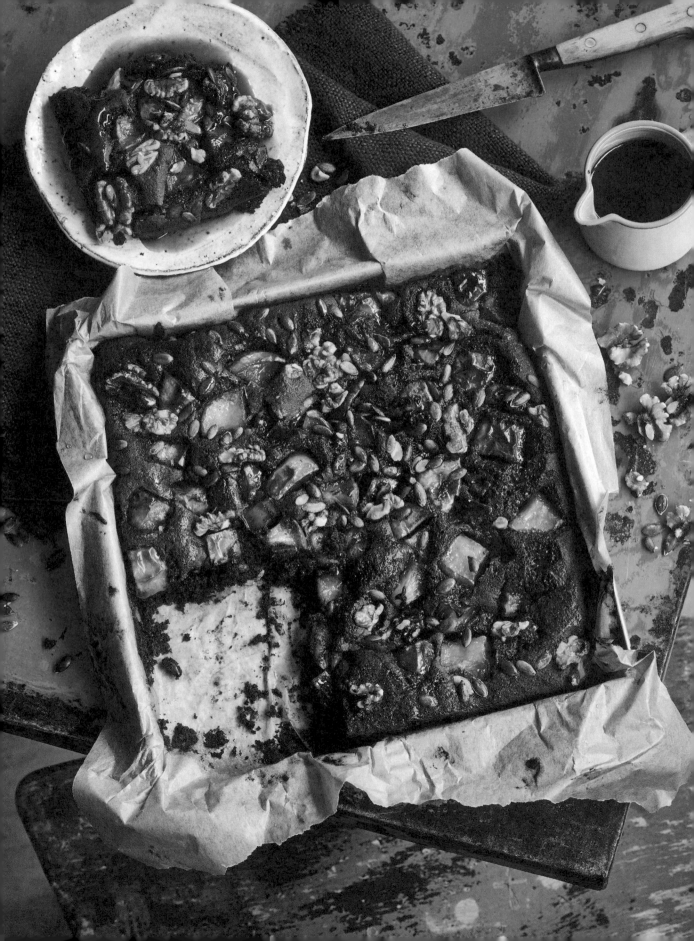

PORTUGUESE TARTS

MAKES **8**	COOKS IN **55 MINS**	DIFFICULTY **5/10**

CAN
BE
GF

vegetable oil, for greasing

3 tbsp plain (all-purpose) flour
or gluten-free flour, for dusting

1 pack ready-to-roll puff pastry

2 tbsp ground cinnamon

for the custard

1 x 400-ml (14-fl oz) can of
coconut milk or 400ml (1½ cups)
soy or oat cream

1 tbsp vanilla extract

240ml (1 cup) non-dairy milk

5 tbsp cornflour (cornstarch)

4 tbsp icing (confectioners') sugar

Preheat your oven to 180°C (350°F) and lightly grease 8 holes of a non-stick muffin tray.

Dust your work surface with a little flour, then roll out the pasty into a large rectangle, about 2mm (1/16in) thick. Sprinkle over the cinnamon, covering all of the pastry.

Tightly roll up the pastry widthways into a log shape, then cut the log into 8 rounds.

Roll each round into a disc, about 10cm (4in) in diameter, then press the rounds into the muffin tray holes, making sure the pastry reaches all the way up the sides.

Bake in the oven for 10 minutes.

Meanwhile, make the custard. Add the coconut milk to a saucepan with the vanilla and place the pan over a low heat. Bring to a simmer.

In a mixing bowl, whisk together the non-dairy milk, cornflour (cornstarch) and icing (confectioners') sugar until smooth.

Add the cornflour mix to the saucepan and mix until it's thick and creamy. I alternate between using a rubber spatula and a whisk to stop lumps from forming. It should take around 5–6 minutes for your custard to thicken up. Turn off the heat once thick.

Remove the pastries from the oven, then use a little spoon to flatten the base of each pastry if it's risen high, making more room for custard.

Spoon the custard into each pastry case, then place the filled tarts back into the oven to colour on top for 15–20 minutes. Be careful not to let them burn.

Once golden on top, remove the tarts from the oven and leave to stand for 10 minutes before removing them from the tray and placing them onto a wire rack to completely cool.

The tarts will keep fresh for 2 days if covered.

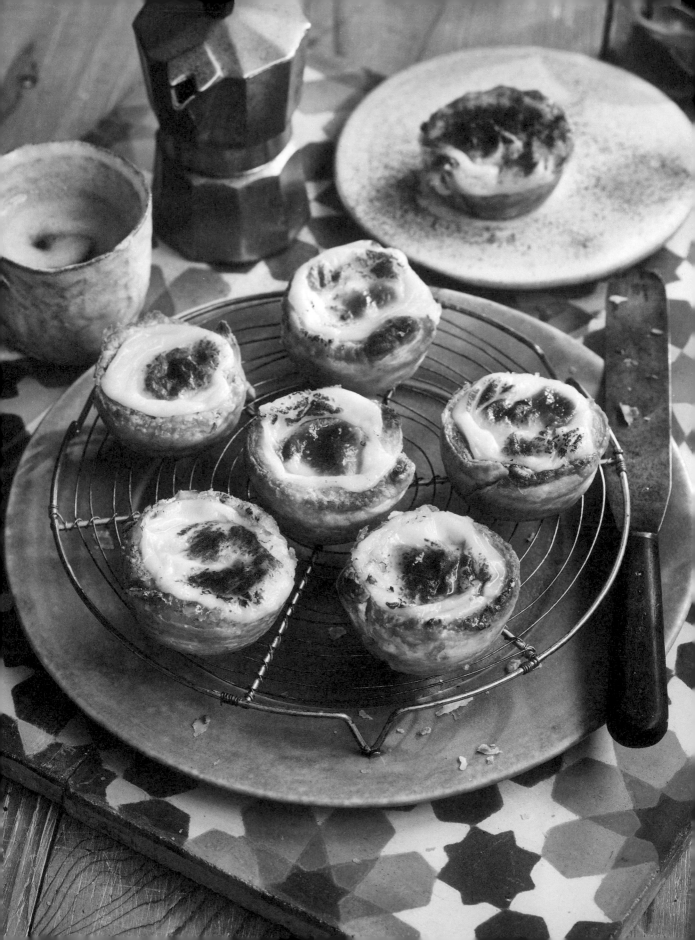

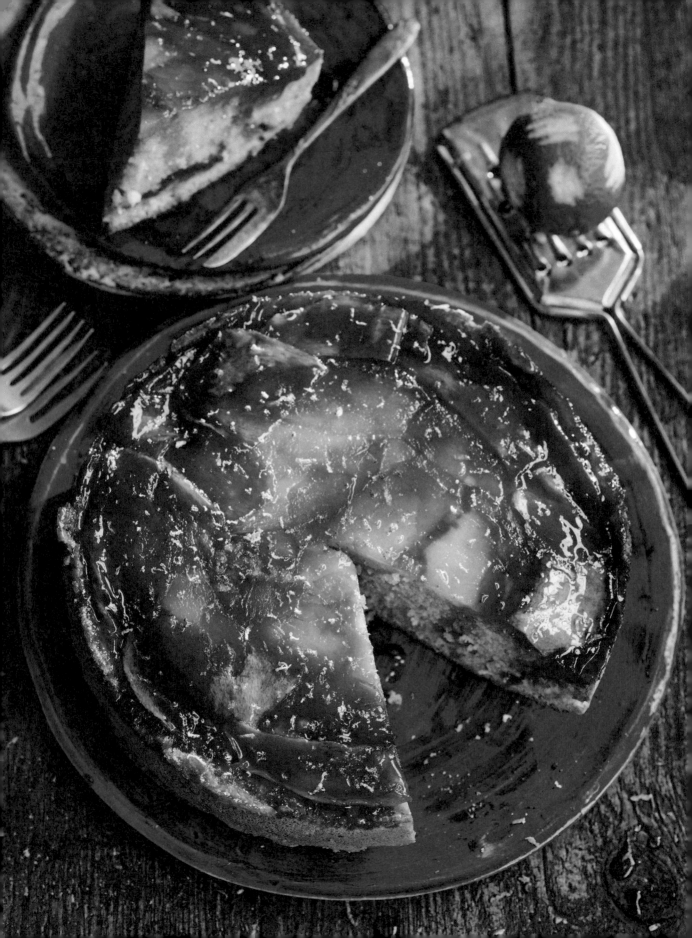

MANGO UPSIDE-DOWN CAKE

I just love upside-down cakes. The mango juices soak into the cake sponge, resulting in a cake like no other.

SERVES 6-8	COOKS IN **75 MINS**	DIFFICULTY **5/10**

for the topping

5 tbsp caster (superfine) sugar

1 tbsp vegan margarine

2 mangoes, peeled and sliced into thin strips

zest of 1 lime, to decorate

for the cake

WET INGREDIENTS

360ml (1½ cup) non-dairy milk

2 tsp vanilla essence

115g (½ cup) vegan margarine, melted

DRY INGREDIENTS

390g (3 cups) plain (all-purpose) flour or gluten-free flour

3 tsp baking powder

pinch sea salt

(300g) 1½ cups caster (superfine) sugar

Preheat your oven to 180°C (350°F) and grease a 23-cm (9-in) diameter loose bottom cake tin. Make sure the bottom seals nice and tightly, or the juices from the fruit will leak out. Place tin on a baking sheet to be safe.

To make the topping, add the caster (superfine) sugar and margarine to a saucepan, place over a low heat and allow them to melt into a caramel. This should take a few minutes; give it a little mix with a spatula from time to time. When the caramel is an amber colour, remove it from the heat – be careful not to leave it too long as it will quickly burn and turn bitter. Be very careful, it will be extremely hot!

Pour the caramel into your cake tin, covering the bottom completely. Neatly lay all the mango strips in the cake tin, on top of the caramel, starting with the edges first and working your way in.

Set the tin aside and quickly make your cake batter.

Combine all the wet ingredients together in a measuring jug.

In a large mixing bowl, sift together the dry ingredients. Pour in the wet mixture and fold together using your spatula in a figure-of-eight motion.

Pour the cake batter directly on top of the mango in the cake tin and give it a little tap on the surface to remove any air pockets.

Pop the cake into the oven on the bottom shelf to bake for 55 minutes, or until a skewer inserted into the cake comes out clean.

Once the cake has cooked, allow it to cool for 5 minutes before turning it out from the tin onto a serving plate. Serve the cake decorated with a little lime zest.

CRÈME CARAMEL

I had to veganize this classic, also known as a flan. This creamy dessert
is so decadent but also very simple to make – give it a try!

MAKES **5**	COOKS IN **60 MINS**	DIFFICULTY **7/10**

for the caramel

200g (1 cup) caster
(superfine) sugar

120ml (½ cup) water

for the custard filling

480ml (2 cups) soy or oat cream

1 tbsp vanilla extract

240ml (1 cup) soy milk

6 tbsp cornflour (cornstarch)

5 tbsp maple syrup (or to taste)

to garnish

fresh mint

Gather together 5 metal dariole moulds or ramekins on a baking sheet.

First, make the caramel. Add the sugar to a saucepan with the water then
place the pan over a low heat. Let the sugar melt down and turn into an
amber-coloured caramel. Don't stir the caramel, just swirl the pan around
to help it mix. Please be very careful when handling the caramel, it will be
super hot.

Pour a couple of tablespoons of caramel into the bottom of each mould/
ramekin. Let the caramel in the moulds completely set and cool at room
temperature before making the filling.

For the filling, add the soy or oat cream to a saucepan with the vanilla
and place the pan over a low heat. Bring to a simmer.

Meanwhile, in a mixing bowl, whisk together the soy milk, cornflour
(cornstarch) and maple syrup until it's smooth.

Add the cornflour mix to the saucepan with the cream and mix until it's thick
and creamy. I alternate between using a rubber spatula and a whisk to stop
lumps from forming. It should take around 5–6 minutes for your custard to
thicken up. Turn off the heat once thick.

Neatly spoon the custard into your moulds and smooth them over using the
back of your spoon. Cover over the tray with cling film (plastic wrap), then
place them into the fridge for at least 6 hours to set.

Before serving, carefully turn the crème caramels out onto individual plates
and garnish with fresh mint.

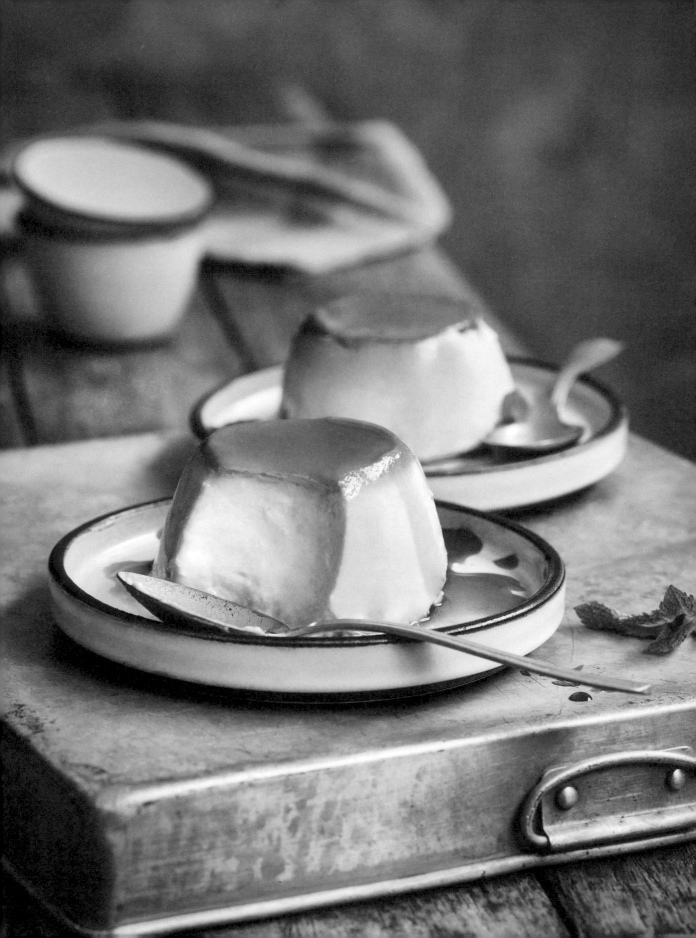

WHOLE ROASTED PINEAPPLES

This is my absolute favourite way to eat pineapple. Beautifully caramelized on the outside and even juicer and sweeter on the inside after roasting.

SERVES **6**	COOKS IN **30 MINS**	DIFFICULTY **3/10**	GF

2 tbsp coconut sugar

2 tsp ground cinnamon

½ tsp cayenne pepper

1 tbsp coconut oil

2 pineapples, peeled

to garnish

toasted coconut flakes

dairy-free ice cream

fresh mint

maple syrup

lime zest

Preheat your oven to 180°C (350°F).

Add the coconut sugar, cinnamon and cayenne pepper to a small bowl and mix together.

Place a large non-stick pan over a medium heat and add the coconut oil. When hot, add the pineapples. Turn the pineapples so that they colour on all sides. Sprinkle over the sugar mixture while they are cooking.

When the pineapples are golden, place them onto a baking sheet, then into the oven for 15–20 minutes.

Once baked, carve the pineapples at the table and serve with toasted coconut flakes, ice cream, fresh mint, a drizzle of maple syrup and a little lime zest.

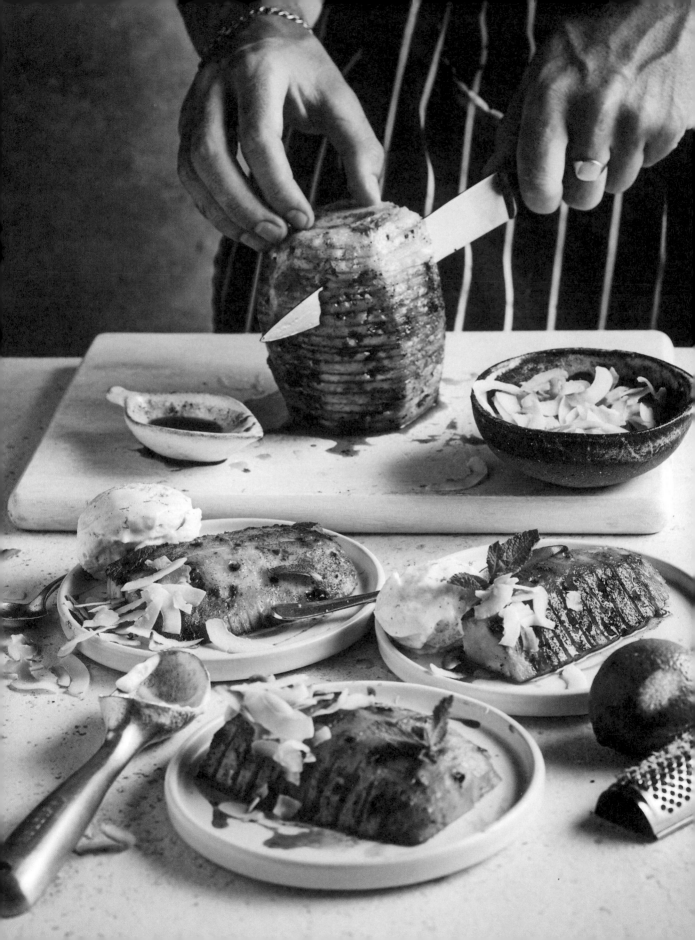

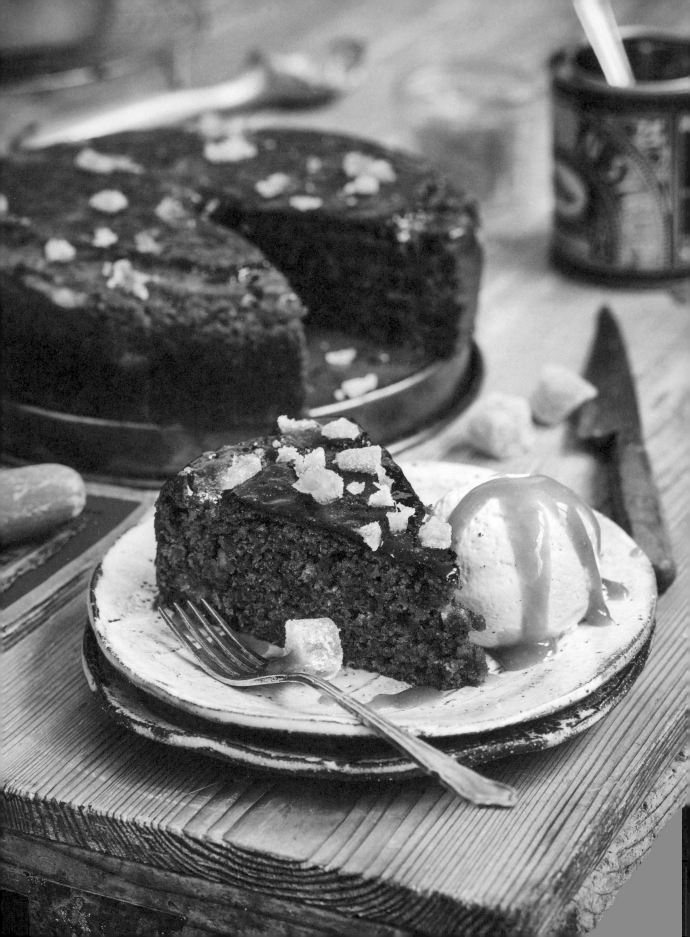

STICKY GINGERBREAD CAKE

| SERVES 6–8 | COOKS IN **90 MINS** | DIFFICULTY **5/10** |

½ ripe banana

240ml (1 cup) non-dairy milk

100g (½ cup) vegan margarine

110g (⅓ cup) treacle

110g (⅓ cup) golden syrup

100g (½ cup) brown sugar

225g (1¾ cups) self-raising flour

1 tsp bicarbonate of soda (baking soda)

2 tsp ground ginger

1 tsp mixed spice

30g (¼ cup) pitted dates, finely chopped

60g (¼ cup) crystallized (candied) ginger, finely chopped, plus a little extra for garnish

serve with

Caramel Sauce (page 210)

non-dairy ice cream

Preheat your oven to 180°C (350°F) and line a 23-cm (9-in) loose-bottom cake tin.

In a mixing bowl, mash together the banana with the milk, until there are very few lumps.

In another bowl, beat the margarine, treacle, golden syrup and brown sugar together until the sugar has dissolved. Sift the flour, bicarbarbonate of soda (baking soda) and spices into the same bowl, then fold until the dry ingredients are fully incorporated.

Add the chopped dates, crystallized (candied) ginger and then the banana and milk mixture. Mix everything together well.

Pour the cake mix into your lined tin, then place it into the oven for 55 minutes.

After 55 minutes of baking, insert a clean skewer into the middle of the cake to see if it's cooked. If it comes out clean, the cake is done; if not, pop it back into the oven for slightly longer.

Once baked, let the cake stand for 15 minutes before carefully turning it out from the cake tin. Let the cake cool completely on a wire rack.

To serve, garnish the cake with some extra crystallized ginger, and serve with Caramel Sauce and ice cream.

LIME PIES

SERVES **5–6** | COOKS IN **35 MINS** | DIFFICULTY **5/10**

CAN
BE
GF

160g (⅔ cup) vegan butter, melted, plus extra for greasing

1 x 250-g (9-oz) pack Lotus Biscoff biscuits or vegan cookies of your choice

for the lime filling

1 x 400-ml (14-fl oz) can coconut milk

2 tbsp fresh lime zest

juice of 2 limes

½ tsp matcha (optional)

280ml (1¼ cups) almond milk

4 tbsp cornflour (cornstarch)

5 tbsp caster (superfine) sugar

to serve

Soft Italian-Style Meringue (page 210)

fresh lime slices

fresh blackberries

Preheat your oven to 180°C (350°F). Lightly grease a 23-cm (9-in) loose-bottom tart tin, or five smaller ones (10cm/4in diameter).

Add the cookies to a food processor and blitz to a fine crumb. While blitzing, add the melted butter. Tip the biscuit mixture into your greased tart tin(s) and use a spoon to compress the mixture to form the biscuit base. Press the mixture up the sides of the tin(s) as well. Smooth out the mixture making sure it's an even layer all over.

Place the tin(s) in the oven to bake until firm for 12 minutes. Remove and allow to cool.

To make the lime filling, gently heat the coconut milk with the lime zest, juice and matcha (if using) in a medium-sized saucepan, over a low heat.

Combine the almond milk, cornflour (cornstarch) and sugar in a bowl, and whisk until completely mixed. When the coconut milk is hot, pour the almond milk mixture into the pan and whisk over the heat until the mix starts to thicken.

Continue to whisk for 2 more minutes or until the mixture is super-thick and custard-like.

Carefully pour the lime filling mixture into the cooled pie case(s). Neatly spread the filling out using an offset palette knife. Then place a layer of clingfilm (plastic wrap) directly over the filling, making sure there are no air pockets. This is important – it stops a skin forming.

Place the pie(s) in the fridge to chill for at least 4 hours before serving.

Prepare your meringue following the method on page 210, spoon it onto the pie(s) and finish with a blow torch or place under a hot grill (broiler) for a minute or so until browned. Add slices of lime and blackberries to serve.

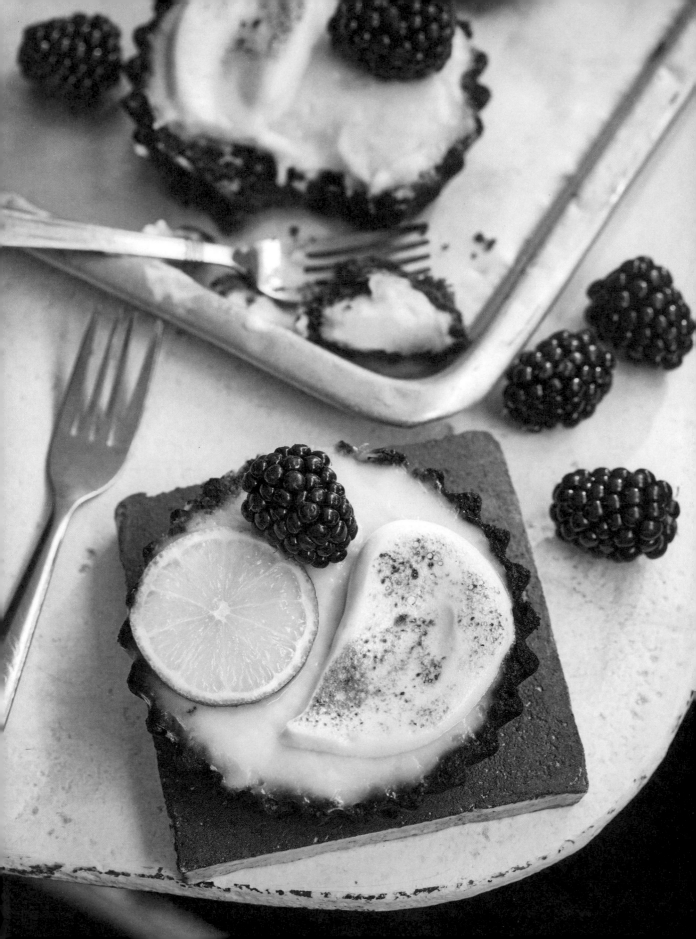

SOFT ITALIAN-STYLE MERINGUE

MAKES APPROX. 2 CUPS

240ml (1 cup) chickpea (garbanzo) water

60g (½ cup) icing (confectioners') sugar

1 tsp vanilla essence

¼ tsp xanthan gum

¼ tsp cream of tartar

Place all the ingredients into a mixing bowl, then using an electric whisk, whisk the ingredients until you have stiff peaks. This should take around 5 minutes.

Pipe the meringue onto cakes, pies or tarts and finish with a blow torch (or place under a hot grill/broiler) for a caramelized flavour.

Alternatively you can bake the meringue in your oven, set at 100°C (220°F) for 4–5 hours.

CARAMEL SAUCE

MAKES APPROX. 2 CUPS

200g (1 cup) caster (superfine) sugar

4 tbsp golden syrup

120ml (½ cup) dairy-free cream, such as soy or oat

115g (½ cup) tbsp vegan margarine

1 tsp vanilla bean paste, or to taste

Add the caster (superfine) sugar and golden syrup to a heavy-based saucepan. Place the pan over a medium heat and allow the sugar to melt to an amber-coloured caramel.

Once melted, take the pan off the heat, then carefully whisk in the cream and margarine.

Once incorporated, place the sauce back over a low heat and stir in the vanilla to taste.

COCONUT CREAM

MAKES APPROX. 1½ CUPS

1 x 400-ml (14-fl oz) can full-fat coconut milk (refrigerated)

3 tbsp icing (confectioners') sugar or sweetener of your choice

1 tsp vanilla extract

Scoop out the thick, creamy coconut milk from the tin, leaving the watery bit behind.

Add the creamy coconut milk to a mixing bowl, along with the icing (confectioners') sugar and vanilla, then whisk with an electric whisk until the mixture is thick and creamy.

Store the cream in your fridge until you need it. It will keep for 2–3 days in an airtight container.

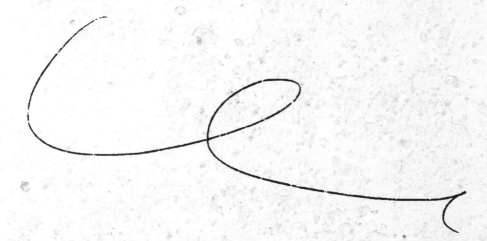

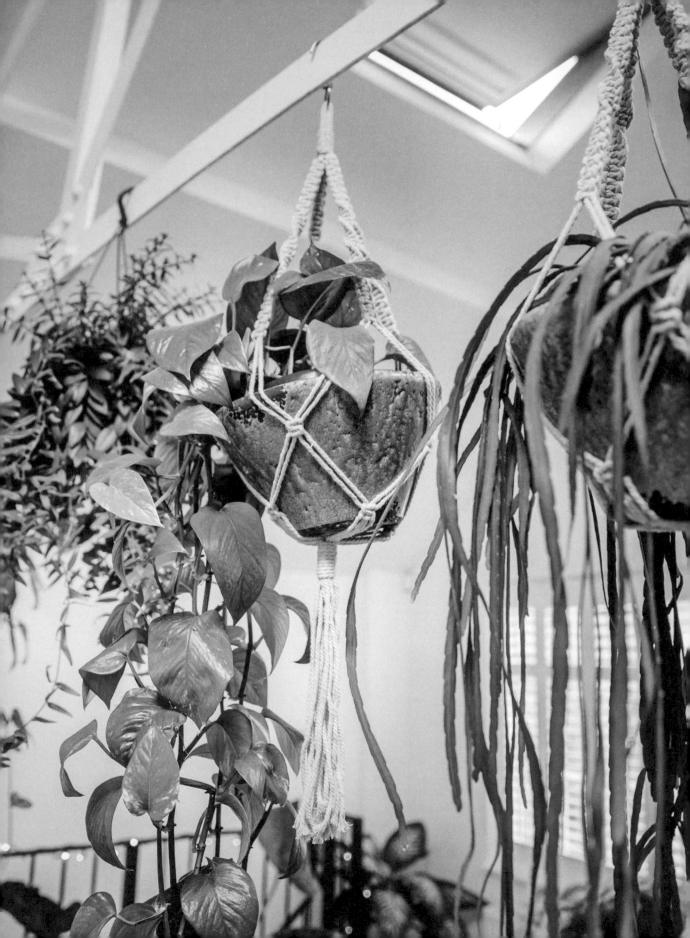

PLATE METHOD

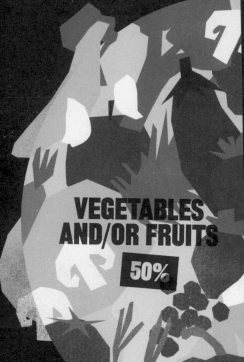
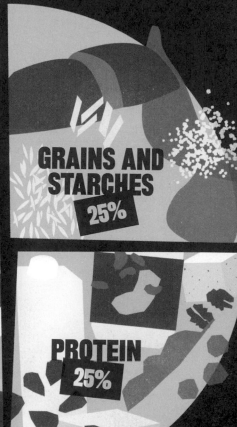

GRAINS AND STARCHES
25%

VEGETABLES AND/OR FRUITS
50%

PROTEIN
25%

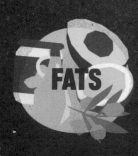

FATS

DAIRY SUBS

EXTRA SUPPLEMENTS

The plate method is an easy visual tool to ensure your meals are nutritionally balanced. Visualize this ratio for a meal whether it's on a plate or in a bowl.

The diagram above simplifies portion sizes and outlines general food groups to include in a nutritionally balanced meal.

TIP: Many of my recipes can be made oil-free, just swap the oil out for a little water when cooking.

feat. @pickuplimes

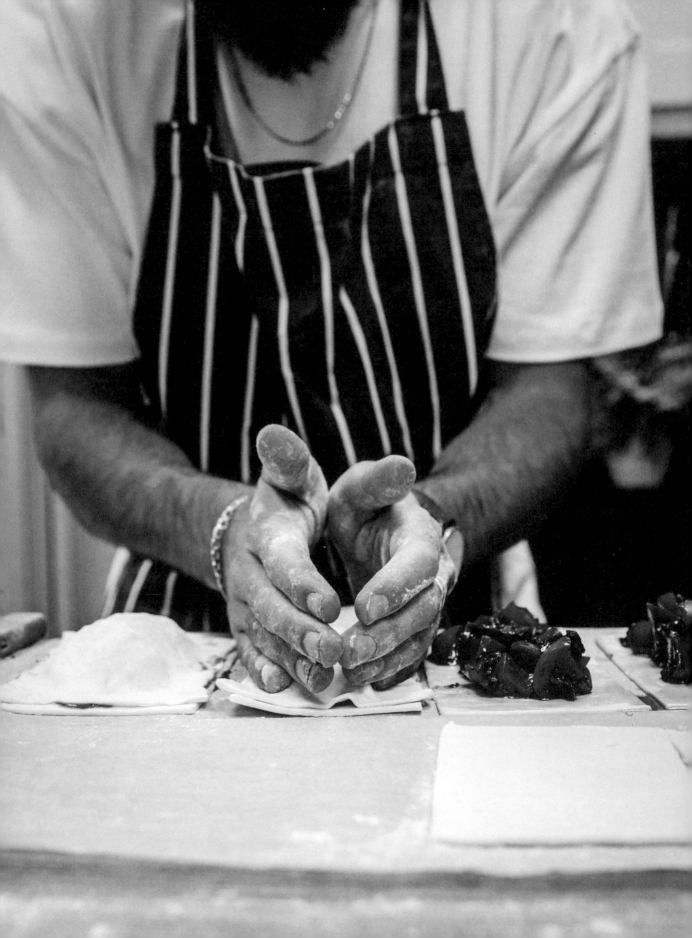

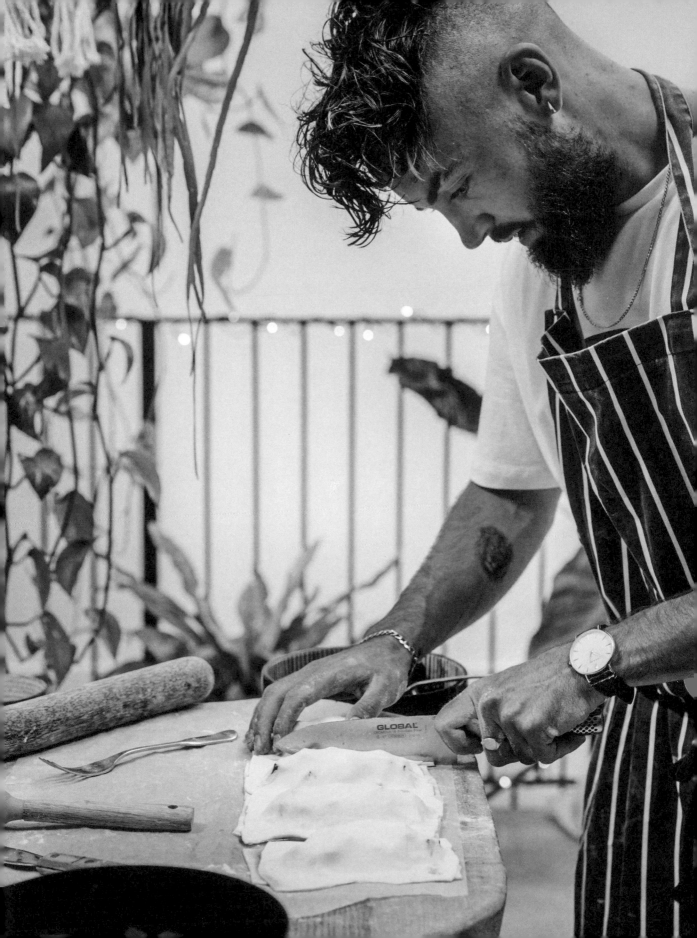

INDEX

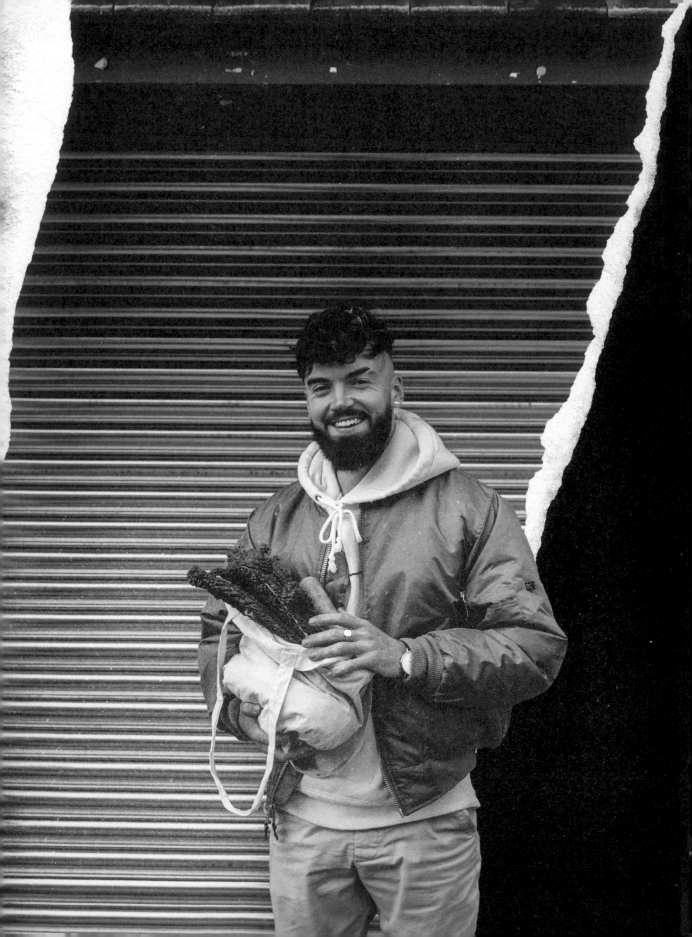

ACKNOWLEDGMENTS

There are so many people to thank – I'm lucky to have a great team around me.

Thanks again to my incredible family – Mum, Dad and sister Charlotte – for all the support. Dad, thanks for helping me test the recipes, and Mum, thanks for eating them! Thanks for all the amazing work you put in behind the scenes working on Avant-Garde Vegan – you're the best!

Thanks Mark Parry and Joe Horner, two dear friends who assisted me greatly during the photoshoot. It was exhausting, but so fun.

Simon Smith, Ashley and Simon #2, thanks so much for all your efforts shooting the food. The pictures look beautiful and it's such a joy working with you. Can't wait for the next one.

Tom Lewis my mate and epic content creator, thanks for all you do working on my videos, helping me create the best content possible and bringing my visions to life.

Zoe, my agent and friend, thanks so much for all your hard work. I couldn't do this without you.

Peter O'Sullivan, thanks so much for smashing the lifestyle pictures and making me look half decent, ha!

Thanks so much White Sky Creative for putting the book together so beautifully.

Quadrille/Hardie Grant, thanks so much for all your hard work making this book happen.

And finally...

Thanks to my incredible supporters for purchasing *Plants Only Kitchen*. It means the world.

Gaz

PUBLISHING DIRECTOR Sarah Lavelle
PROJECT EDITOR Amy Christian
DESIGN White Sky Creative
FOOD PHOTOGRAPHER Simon Smith
LIFESTYLE PHOTOGRAPHER Peter O'Sullivan
PROP STYLING Luis Peral, with Gaz Oakley
FOOD STYLING Gaz Oakley
PRODUCTION CONTROLLER Nikolaus Ginelli
HEAD OF PRODUCTION Stephen Lang

Published in 2020 by Quadrille, an imprint of Hardie Grant Publishing

Quadrille
52–54 Southwark Street
London SE1 1UN
quadrille.com

Cataloguing in Publication Data: a catalogue record for this book is available from the British Library.

ISBN 978 1 78713 498 0

Printed in China

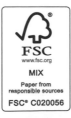

FSC
www.fsc.org
MIX
Paper from
responsible sources
FSC® C020056